SpringerWienNewYork

Acta Neurochirurgica
Supplements

Editor: H.-J. Steiger

Trends in Neurovascular Surgery

Edited by

T. Tsukahara, L. Regli, D. Hänggi, B. Turowski, H.-J. Steiger

Acta Neurochirurgica
Supplement 112

SpringerWienNewYork

Tetsuya Tsukahara
Department of Neurosurgery, National Hospital Organization, Kyoto Medical Center, 1-1 Mukaihata-cho, Fukakusa, Fushimi-ku, 612–8555 Kyoto, Japan
ttsukaha@kyotolan.hosp.go.jp

Luca Regli
Department of Neurosurgery, Rudolf Magnus Institute of Neuroscience, University Medical Center, Heidelberglaan 100, GA 3508, Utrecht, The Netherlands
l.regli@umcutrecht.nl

Daniel Hänggi
Department of Neurosurgery, Heinrich Heine University, Moorenstraße 5, 40225 Düsseldorf, Germany
daniel.haenggi@med.uni-duesseldorf.de

Bernd Turowski
Department of Neurosurgery, Heinrich Heine University, Moorenstraße 5, 40225 Düsseldorf, Germany
bernd.turowski@uni-duesseldorf.de

Hans-Jakob Steiger
Department of Neurosurgery, Heinrich Heine University, Moorenstraße 5, 40225 Düsseldorf, Germany
steiger@uni-duesseldorf.de

Printed in Germany
SpringerWienNewYork is part of Springer Science+Business Media
springer.at

Typesetting: SPI, Pondichery, India

Printed on acid-free and chlorine-free bleached paper
SPIN: 80022360

Library of Congress Control Number: 2011928406

With 117 (partly coloured) Figures

ISSN 0065-1419
ISBN 978-3-7091-0660-0 e-ISBN 978-3-7091-0661-7
DOI: 10.1007/978-3-7091-0661-7
SpringerWienNewYork

Preface

The *European-Japanese Joint Conferences for Stroke Surgery* were initiated in 2001 by Prof. Y. Sakurai, Sendai, and Prof. Y. Yonekawa, Zürich, under the name the *Swiss-Japanese Joint Conference*. The first meeting in Zürich was dedicated to the management of subarachnoid hemorrhage and unruptured aneurysms. The renewed interest in bypass surgery and other technical aspects of neurovascular disease generated the need for a regular platform dedicated to surgical and endovascular aspects of stroke treatment and stroke prevention. The second meeting was also organized in Zürich two years later. The third meeting, now under the name of the *European-Japanese Joint Conference for Stroke Surgery*, was held in 2006 in conjunction with the 70th Anniversary of the *Neurochirurgische Universitätsklinik Zürich* founded by Prof. Krayenbühl. The fourth meeting was organized for the first time outside Switzerland and was held in Helsinki, Finland, in 2008, with Prof. Hernesniemi as the congress president.

The fifth *European-Japanese Joint Conference for Stroke Surgery* was held from 8 to 11 July 2010 in Düsseldorf, Germany. The main topics of the conference were the management of cerebral and ventricular hemorrhage, extra-intracranial bypass surgery, surgical and endovascular treatment of cervical and intracranial arterial occlusive disease, and embolization and microsurgery of AVM and dural AV fistulas. Sessions for free topics completed the program. In order to strengthen the focus on upcoming new trends, open invitation for submission of abstracts was used to constitute the majority of the program. The resulting meeting fulfilled the expectations of the organizers in that a number of emerging concepts were presented and discussed. The actual volume presents the resulting original papers of the meeting.

Kyoto — Tetsuya Tsukahara
Utrecht — Luca Regli
Düsseldorf — Daniel Hänggi
Düsseldorf — Bernd Turowski
Düsseldorf — Hans-Jakob Steiger

Contents

Management of Cerebral and Ventricular Hemorrhage

Endoscopic Intra-Hematomal Evacuation of Intracerebral Hematomas – A Suitable Technique for Patients with Coagulopathies

Berk Orakcioglu, Y. Uozumi, and A. Unterberg

Abstract *Objectives*: To describe an endoscopic technique to evacuate acute intracerebral hemorrhage (ICH) using the balanced suction-irrigation method in patients with intrinsic or iatrogenic coagulopathies.

Methods: We report on our early experience with four patients with atypical ICH related to intrinsic and iatrogenic coagulopathies. In all patients, an endoscopic hematoma evacuation was performed using a navigated burrhole approach. The entry site and trajectory were planned according to the long axis of the hematoma.

Results: Every operation was carried out with the aid of neuronavigation. Gross total removal of the hematoma was not intended as first line, especially if eloquent areas could be avoided. Intra-hematomal evacuation leaving minimal hematoma remnants was performed in three of four patients. We report hematoma removal rates of approximately 90%. In all patients, a significant hematoma reduction was achieved, although residues were tolerated to limit neurological damage. No re-hemorrhage was observed.

Conclusion: The endoscopic technique with the aid of neuronavigation may be an appropriate method to safely evacuate ICH in the acute stage in patients with intrinsic or iatrogenic coagulopathies.

Keywords ICH · Endoscopy · Balanced suction-irrigation technique · Antiplatelet · Warfarin · Coagulopathy

B. Orakcioglu (✉)
Department of Neurosurgery, Ruprecht Karl University, Heidelberg, Germany and
Department of Neurosurgery, University Hospital Heidelberg, Im Neuenheimer Feld 400, 69120 Heidelberg, Germany
e-mail: berk.orakcioglu@med.uni-heidelberg.de

Y. Uozumi and A. Unterberg
Department of Neurosurgery, Ruprecht Karl University, Heidelberg, Germany

Introduction

Ever since the STICH trial, neurosurgeons have had reasonable concerns about whether to evacuate an intracerebral hematoma (ICH) or not [7]. Neither this randomized controlled study nor the following meta-analyses have proved surgery to be beneficial in the acute stage [8]. However, refined endoscopic techniques have become available and recent reports show good results with this method in comparison to the conventional operations [11]. Due to small patient numbers and retrospective designs, other studies with promising endoscopic methods have also failed to argue definitively for an operation [1, 9, 12]. In light of an older and debated study that demonstrated a significant benefit of endoscopic hematoma evacuation compared to conservative treatment, a reevaluation of these methods seems justified.

Patients at risk for early re-hemorrhage or progressive hemorrhage, such as patients with intrinsic or iatrogenic coagulopathies, are usually treated conservatively because surgery may place them at even higher risk of hematoma growth and subsequently worse outcome. Others have reported that the pre- or perioperative administration of rFVIIa resulted in minimal residual or recurrent hematoma volume and may be an important adjunct to surgery in patients with intracerebral hemorrhage [16]. Pure systemic delivery of rFVIIa, although a promising medical treatment, failed to prove clinical benefit in the FAST trial [6]. Hematoma growth was counteracted, but medical complications related to thrombosis and cardiovascular events diluted this positive neurological effect with regard to outcome. On the other hand, limited tissue damage using endoscopic methods has the potential to safely evacuate parts of an ICH and thereby reduce secondary neuron damage. Although endoscopes are proving to be increasingly useful for maximizing surgical efficacy while minimizing invasiveness, some doubts remain about their ability to allow for controlled intraoperative hemostasis and re-hemorrhage prevention. New techniques that have been introduced by others are studied in this small series of patients with coagulation abnormalities [9, 11].

T. Tsukahara et al. (eds.), *Trends in Neurovascular Surgery*, Acta Neurochirurgica Supplementum, Vol. 112,
DOI: 10.1007/978-3-7091-0661-7_1, © Springer-Verlag/Wien 2011

Methods

The endoscope used for surgery is rigid, measuring 0° and 2.7 mm in diameter (Richard Wolf GmbH, Knittlingen, Germany). The Nagasaka combined irrigation-coagulation suction cannula (Fujita Medical Instruments, Tokyo, Japan) was used to evacuate the hematomas within a transparent sheath (Neuroport, Olympus, Tokyo, Japan) that is used as the working channel to the core of the hematoma positioned along its long axis. For accurate preoperative planning, a thin-sliced CT scan was obtained immediately before surgery. This CT was used for neuronavigation with the Brainlab (BrainLab AG, Feldkirchen, Germany) system. Entry site and trajectory plans were prepared for each patient in order to avoid eloquent brain regions to reduce approach-related morbidity. If more than one plausible entry site existed, the less eloquent track was chosen, even though the hematoma may have extended less superficially.

Results

Patient characteristics are presented in Table 1. One patient presented with a left frontal lobar hematoma after aspirin use. Another patient was treated with warfarin and had an INR of 4.3 on presentation. A patient with trauma-associated ICH had a coagulopathy due to chronic alcoholism, and another patient harbored an atypical right temporo-parietal ICH due to sinus-vein thrombosis. He received continuous i.v. heparin with a prolonged activated partial thromboplastin time (APTT). After sequential proof of progressive hematoma growth, an endoscopic intra-hematomal evacuation was performed in order to limit tissue damage. In summary, all patients either received anticoagulants ($n=3$) or suffered from intrinsic coagulopathies ($n=1$). Every operation was carried out with the aid of neuronavigation. Gross total removal of the hematoma was not intended as first line, especially if eloquent areas could be avoided. Consequently, we report hematoma removal rates of approximately 80–90%, which are less than previously reported elsewhere [10]. Mean operation times were 58 ± 12 min from skin incision to closure. Trajectory and entry site planning cost approximately 5 min of additional preoperative time, but clearly enhanced safety and accuracy to conform to the optimum trajectory. As a primary goal for surgery in this special selection of potentially complicated patients, aggressive evacuation of all hematoma components was avoided. Intra-hematomal evacuation leaving minimal hematoma remnants was performed in three of four cases. During the operation, minor bleedings were sufficiently dealt with using the multifunctional Nagasaki instrument. Finally, burr holes were sealed with bone dust after dural closure. We did not observe any postoperative re-hemorrhage, CSF or wound infection, neurological worsening or hydrocephalus.

Table 1 Patient characteristics

Case	Age	Location	Etiology	Volume (mL)	Neurological deficit	Evacuation rate (% of intended volume)	Postoperative volume (mL)	GCS preoperative	Best GCS postoperative	Rebleeding
1	45	Left frontal, cortical	INR 4.3	71	Hemiparesis, global aphasia	>90	6.5	15	15	No
2	66	Right fronto-temporal, cortical, trauma related	Chronic alcohol abuse, liver dysfunction	108	Hemiparesis	80	20	7	15	No
3	71	Right fronto-parietal, cortical, IVH	Aspirin	152	Hemiparesis	>95	7	10	15	No
4	62	Right temporo-occipital, cortical	Sinus-vein thrombosis, i.v. heparin	82	Hemianopia, hemiparesis	>85	13	8	15	No

GCS Glasgow coma score, *INR* international normalized ratio, *IVH* intraventricular hemorrhage

Case Illustration

A 71-year-old woman was transferred to our hospital because of left-sided hemiparesis. On admission, her Glasgow Coma Scale (GCS) score was 15. A computed tomographic scan of the head revealed right frontoparietal ICH with a moderate space-occupying effect. She reported daily aspirin use for unspecific reasons. After neurological deterioration and drowsiness (GCS 10), a repeat spiral CCT showed hematoma progression, the volume of which was estimated to be 151.5 mL (Fig. 1a) using the a*b*c/2 method described elsewhere [5]. Moderate ventricular involvement with progressive clinical signs of hydrocephalus had developed within 12h of onset (Fig. 1b). These image sets were fused with the BrainLab neuronavigation system (BrainLab AG, Feldkirchen, Germany). According to the long axis of the hematoma, an entry site and optimum trajectory were drawn preoperatively sparing eloquent areas (Fig. 2). Endoscopic evacuation of the hematoma was performed with the patient under general anesthesia with the head fixed in a three-pin headholder. Using the intra-hematomal evacuation technique, no hemorrhaging occurred. The balanced irrigation-suction technique made complete ventricular clearance of all solid hematoma components possible. Complete evacuation of the indented hematoma parts and IVH was accomplished. Postoperative computed tomography confirmed the complete removal of the hematoma (Fig. 3). As expected, the previously ascertained left hemiparesis persisted, but the level of consciousness improved to a Glasgow Coma Scale score of 15 at postoperative day 2. Because of this, the patient was transferred back to her primary hospital on the second day after hematoma removal. Within 2 months after the operation she regained some motor function on her left side, scored 7 on the extended Glasgow Outcome Scale (eGOS), and is otherwise neurologically intact. Hydrocephalus never occurred postoperatively.

Discussion

Secondary neuronal injury after ICH is possibly linked to the existence of a "perihemorrhagic penumbra" [2, 3, 13, 15], which is mainly related to hematoma size. Therefore hematoma reduction has been a surgical target ever since,

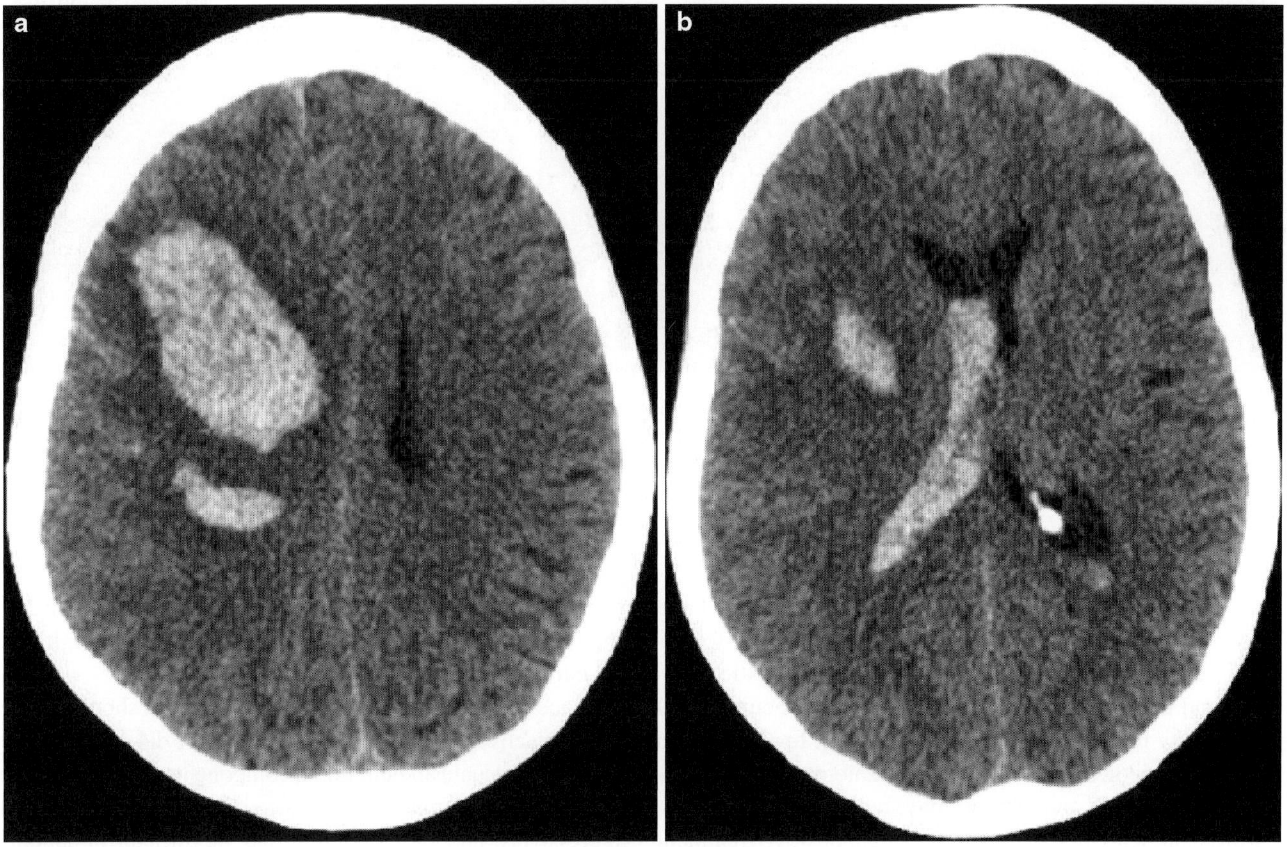

Fig. 1 Preoperative CT-scan demonstrating a large right-frontal ICH and a smaller right central ICH with moderate displacement of midline structures (**a**) and deeper ICH components and unilateral ventricular hemorrhage (**b**)

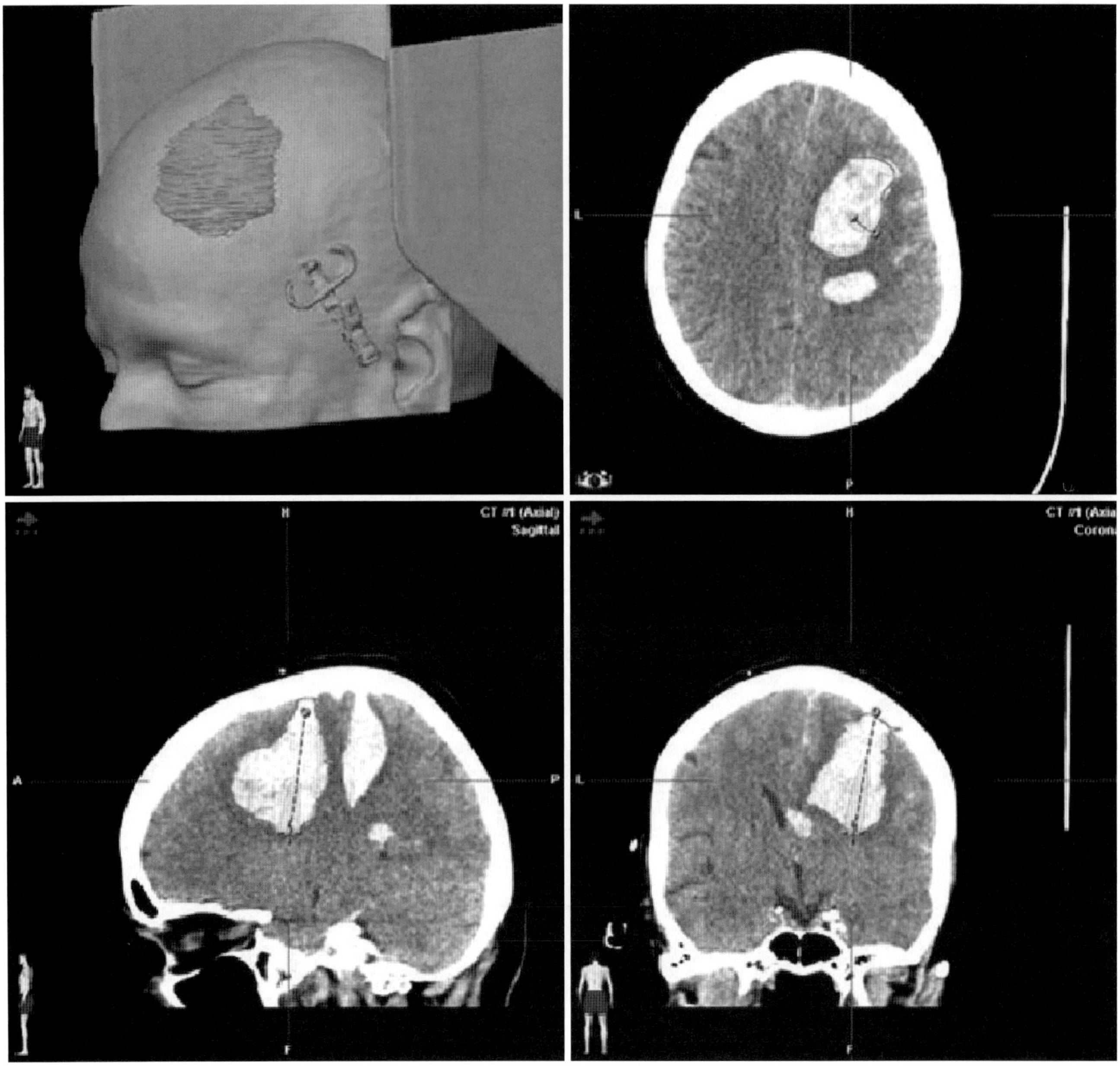

Fig. 2 BrainLab (BrainLab AG Feldkirchen, Germany) screenshot of the preoperative entry-site and trajectory plan. ICH is seen on the *right side* of the figure (opposite to the CT-scan), which represents the anatomical right side. Note that the centrally located hematoma appears to be somewhat isolated in the sagittal plane and was not intended for ICH-evacuation because of high surgical morbidity

although the superiority of surgical interventions of whichever kind has so far not been statistically proven in large trials [7]. Not withstanding, ICH surgery is practiced worldwide, and the technological advances of diagnostic measures and therapeutic options seem to improve neurological outcome by reducing invasiveness [1, 9–12]. In comparison to the best medical treatment, open craniotomy and microscopic hematoma evacuation may represent a relatively harmful surgical approach that may dilute positive treatment effects. Furthermore, the use of neuronavigation during ICH evacuation has not been reported in the literature and may potentially reduce surgical morbidity, as seen for other neurosurgical procedures [4]. Therefore, we aimed to investigate surgical ICH patients with atypical hematomas at high risk for intraoperative or rehemorrhage.

Since preservation of neurological function should be the main objective of any surgical procedure, we did not primarily intend to evacuate all hematoma components maximally. The margins of the hematoma may bleed diffusely once handled aggressively, and cautherization may be difficult in patients with documented antiplatelet activity, warfarin use or any other coagulopathy. The authors believe that these surgical

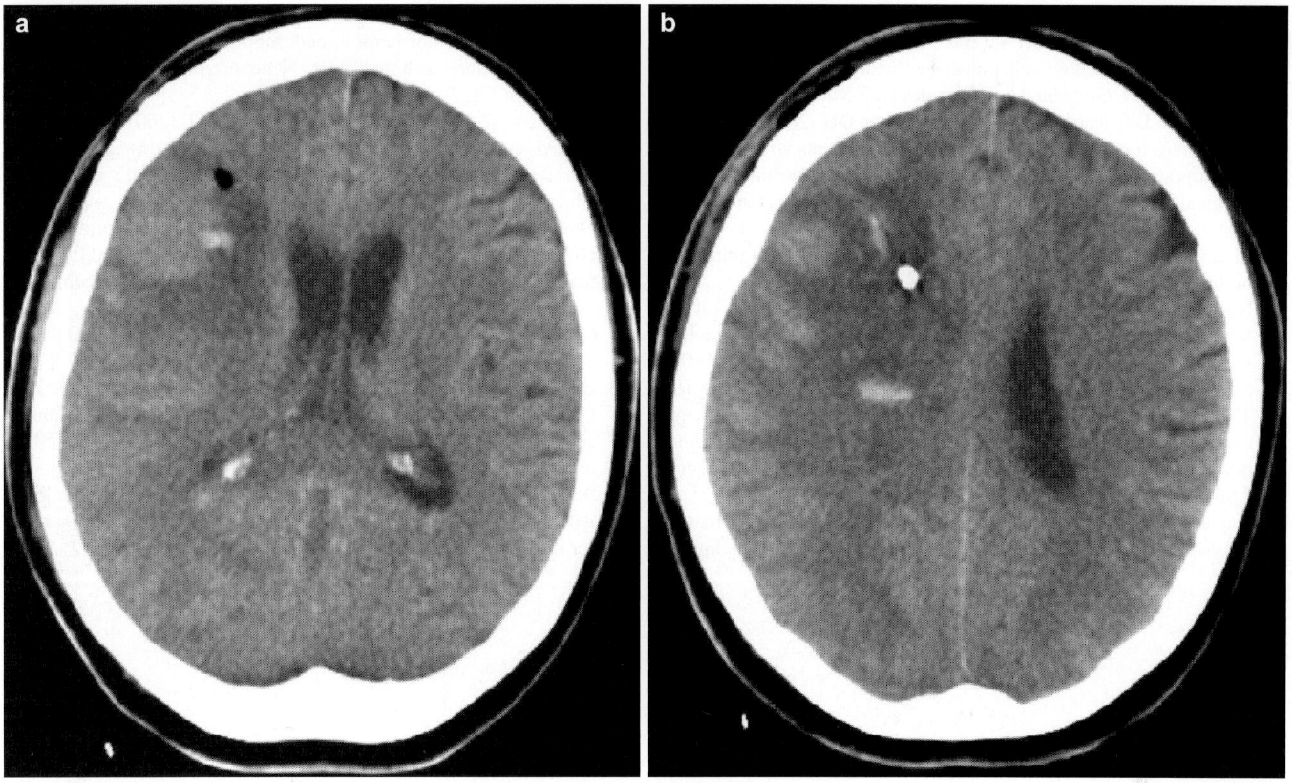

Fig. 3 Representative post-operative CCT (day 1) proving almost complete removal of the intended ICH (**a**, **b**) and gross ventricular clearance

steps are likely to increase surgical morbidity. Therefore, we performed intra-hematomal evacuations using an endoscopic burr hole approach, which avoided intraoperative hemorrhaging, even though small hematoma remnants were tolerated in eloquent areas (Fig. 3). This operative ulterior motive is supported by unpublished experimental data suggesting that the secondary neuronal injury measured by cerebral blood flow, $P_{br}O_2$ and microdialysis increase with hematoma expansion [14]. According to the authors', small hematomas do not negatively influence the perihemorrhagic metabolism and therefore do not need to be addressed aggressively.

Another aspect to enhance safety in hematoma evacuation is the use of neuronavigation. To the authors' knowledge, this has not been reported in the pertinent literature up to date. Most likely this is related to the nature of ICH surgery, which is most often performed when neuronavigation resources are limited. Our limited experience suggests that neuronavigation will increase surgical accuracy, reduce morbidity and shorten operation times.

In conclusion, endoscopic navigation-aided approaches to atypical ICH with concomitant anticoagulation use or intrinsic coagulopathies may represent a less traumatic surgical option if gross hematoma removal is not the primary goal of the treating surgeon. Consequently, the relevance of such a surgical procedure should be evaluated in larger randomized trials.

Acknowledgment The authors specially thank Dr. T. Nagasaka, who introduced the endoscopic balanced irrigation-suction technique with a multifunctional suction cannula to the Department of Neurosurgery at Heidelberg.

Conflict of interest statement We declare that we have no conflict of interest.

References

1. Bakshi A, Banerji AK (2004) Neuroendoscope-assisted evacuation of large intracerebral hematomas: introduction of a new, minimally invasive technique. Preliminary report. Neurosurg Focus 16:e9
2. Carhuapoma JR, Wang PY, Beauchamp NJ, Keyl PM, Hanley DF, Barker PB (2000) Diffusion-weighted MRI and proton MR spectroscopic imaging in the study of secondary neuronal injury after intracerebral hemorrhage. Stroke 31:726–732
3. Hemphill JC 3rd, Morabito D, Farrant M, Manley GT (2005) Brain tissue oxygen monitoring in intracerebral hemorrhage. Neurocrit Care 3:260–270
4. Iseki H, Nakamura R, Muragaki Y, Suzuki T, Chernov M, Hori T, Takakura K (2008) Advanced computer-aided intraoperative technologies for information-guided surgical management of gliomas: Tokyo Women's Medical University experience. Minim Invasive Neurosurg 51:285–291
5. Kothari MD, Joseph P, Broderick MD, William G, Barsan MD, Laura R, Sauerbeck RN, Mario Zuccarello MD, Jane Khoury MS (1996) The ABCs of measuring intracerebral hemorrhage volumes. Stroke 27:1304–1305

6. Mayer SA, Brun NC, Begtrup K, Broderick J, Davis S, Diringer MN, Skolnick BE, Steiner T (2005) Recombinant activated factor VII for acute intracerebral hemorrhage. N Engl J Med 352:777–785
7. Mendelow AD, Gregson BA, Fernandes HM, Murray GD, Teasdale GM, Hope DT, Karimi A, Shaw MD, Barer DH (2005) Early surgery versus initial conservative treatment in patients with spontaneous supratentorial intracerebral haematomas in the International Surgical Trial in Intracerebral Haemorrhage (STICH): a randomised trial. Lancet 365:387–397
8. Mendelow AD, Unterberg A (2007) Surgical treatment of intracerebral haemorrhage. Curr Opin Crit Care 13:169–174
9. Nagasaka T, Inao S, Ikeda H, Tsugeno M, Okamoto T (2008) Inflation-deflation method for endoscopic evacuation of intracerebral haematoma. Acta Neurochir (Wien) 150:685–690, discussion 690
10. Nagasaka T, Tsugeno M, Ikeda H, Okamoto T, Inao S, Wakabayashi T Early recovery and better evacuation rate in neuroendoscopic surgery for spontaneous intracerebral hemorrhage using a multifunctional cannula: preliminary study in comparison with craniotomy. J Stroke Cerebrovasc Dis
11. Nagasaka T, Tsugeno M, Ikeda H, Okamoto T, Takagawa Y, Inao S, Wakabayashi T (2009) Balanced irrigation-suction technique with a multifunctional suction cannula and its application for intraoperative hemorrhage in endoscopic evacuation of intracerebral hematomas: technical note. Neurosurgery 65(4):E826–E827, discussion E827
12. Nishihara T, Morita A, Teraoka A, Kirino T (2007) Endoscopy-guided removal of spontaneous intracerebral hemorrhage: comparison with computer tomography-guided stereotactic evacuation. Childs Nerv Syst 23:677–683
13. Orakcioglu B, Becker K, Sakowitz OW, Herweh C, Kohrmann M, Huttner HB, Steiner T, Unterberg A, Schellinger PD (2008) MRI of the perihemorrhagic zone in a rat ICH model: effect of hematoma evacuation. Neurocrit Care 8(3):448–455
14. Orakcioglu et al. (2010) Conference proceedings, ICH, Palm Springs 2010
15. Qureshi AI, Ali Z, Suri MF, Shuaib A, Baker G, Todd K, Guterman LR, Hopkins LN (2003) Extracellular glutamate and other amino acids in experimental intracerebral hemorrhage: an in vivo microdialysis study. Crit Care Med 31:1482–1489
16. Sutherland CS, Hill MD, Kaufmann AM, Silvaggio JA, Demchuk AM, Sutherland GR (2008) Recombinant factor VIIa plus surgery for intracerebral hemorrhage. Can J Neurol Sci 35:567–572

The Prediction of 30-Day Mortality and Functional Outcome in Spontaneous Intracerebral Hemorrhage with Secondary Ventricular Hemorrhage: A Score Comparison

Marco Stein, Marcus Luecke, Matthias Preuss, Wolfram Scharbrodt, Aeasndr Joedicke, and Matthias F. Oertel

Abstract The original ICH (oICH) score was tested in different populations and showed good accuracy in the prediction of outcome and 30-day mortality after spontaneous ICH. The oICH was developed to stratify patients with all types of spontaneous intracerebral hemorrhage (SICH). Several modifications of the oICH score exist in the literature.

In the current study, we tested the oICH score, two modified ICH scores, and the IVH score on a cohort of 171 patients with SICH and mandatory secondary intraventricular hemorrhage (IVH). Receiver-operating characteristic (ROC) curves were plotted, and the areas under the curves (AUC) were calculated for each score.

The calculated AUCs for the prediction of 30-day mortality in the cohort were 0.736, 0.816, 0.805, and 0.836 for the original ICH, the mICH-A, the mICH-B, and the new IVH score, respectively. The best AUC for functional outcome was observed for the mICH-B score (0.823). For the mICH-A and the IVH score, an AUC of 0.811 was calculated.

The scores that include the quantification of IVH or the grading of hydrocephalus show good accuracy in the prediction of 30-day mortality and functional outcome at 6 months in SICH with secondary IVH.

Keywords Intracerebral hemorrhage · Intraventricular hemorrhage · Hydrocephalus · ICH score

M. Stein (✉), M. Preuss, W. Scharbrodt, and M.F. Oertel
Department of Neurosurgery, University Hospital Giessen-Marburg, Klinikstrasse 29, 35385 Giessen, Germany
e-mail: dr.stein@email.de

M. Luecke
Department of Neurosurgery, Asklepios Hospital Altona, Klinikstrasse 29, 35385 Giessen, Germany

A. Joedicke
Department of Neurosurgery, Vivantes Hospital Neukölln, Rudower Straße 48, 12351 Berlin, Germany

Introduction

Several scores are known to predict survival and functional outcome in spontaneous intracerebral hemorrhage [2, 7, 9, 13, 15]. Currently, none of these scores has been established in clinical routine for risk stratification of SICH.

The first easy-to-use prediction score for SICH was introduced by Hemphill et al. in 2001 (oICH score) [9]. The oICH score was developed on the basis of independent predictors for 30-day mortality from a retrospective chart review. The score was tested on different populations and showed good predictive value for outcome and mortality [2, 3, 6, 7, 10]. In previous studies, SICH with secondary intraventricular hemorrhage (IVH) was associated with high 30-day mortality rates and unfavorable functional outcome [16].

In 2006, Godoy et al. [7] developed two scores in a modification of the oICH score and compared them with the oICH score. Both modified ICH scores (mICH-A and mICH-B) included the Graeb score, which stratified the intraventricular extension of a hemorrhage.

The role of hydrocephalus in the prediction of outcome is controversial. Hydrocephalus was found to be a predictor of 30-day mortality in some studies [4, 12]. Acute obstructive hydrocephalus in IVH should be treated by the insertion of an external ventricular drain (EVD) [1, 5]. However, up to now no randomized trial has shown a benefit after EVD implantation. The first score to include a categorization of hydrocephalus together with clinical parameters was the IVH score [14].

The aim of this study was to test the accuracy of the different scores on a large cohort of patients with SICH and secondary IVH.

Materials and Methods

A total of 171 patients with the diagnosis of deep-seated intracerebral hematoma and secondary IVH were studied. All patients were admitted to the Department of Neurosurgery of the University Hospital Giessen.

DOI: 10.1007/978-3-7091-0661-7_2, © Springer-Verlag/Wien 2011

Inclusion criteria were the confirmation of SICH and secondary IVH by computerized tomography (CT) and patient age of 18–90 years.

All included patients received at least one external ventricular drain (EVD) to relieve obstructive hydrocephalus. All EVDs were placed in the first 24 h after ictus at our department after the initial CT scan had been reviewed.

Patients with traumatic hemorrhage, ischemic stroke, brain tumor, subarachnoid hemorrhage due to aneurysm or malformation, infratentorial origin of hemorrhage, SICH spreading into the brainstem, strict lobar hematoma, and therapeutic anticoagulation were excluded. Decompressive craniotomy and evacuation of the hematoma were also defined as exclusion criteria.

The first CT scan after ictus before EVD placement was reviewed. Hematoma volume was determined by the ABC/2 method [11]. IVH was graded according to the Graeb scale [8]. For the grading of hydrocephalus we used our own hydrocephalus grading system, which has been published elsewhere [14].

The following scores were compared: the original ICH score (oICH) [9], modified ICH-A and ICH-B score (mICH-A and mICH-B score) [7], and the IVH score. The components of the IVH score were published elsewhere [14].

To estimate the accuracy of each score, the area under the curve (AUC) was calculated using the receiver-operator-characteristic (ROC) method (Fig. 1).

Thirty-day mortality and functional outcome were determined 6 months after ictus.

Good functional outcome was defined as mRS ≤ 3 and bad functional outcome as mRS ≥ 4.

All statistical analyses were computed with the SPSS System 17.0 for Windows (SPSS Inc., Chicago, IL).

Results

A total of 171 patients with deep-seated intracerebral hematoma and secondary IVH who were admitted to our department between January 1995 and July 2008 were reviewed. Ten patients were excluded because of missing follow-up or missing the initial CT scan.

The observed 30-day mortality was 28.6%. Six months after ictus, only 17.4% of the patients showed a favorable functional outcome (mRS ≤ 3).

The baseline characteristics of the cohort are presented in Table 1.

Comparison of the Scores

The highest area under the curve (AUC) for predicting 30-day mortality was observed for the secondary IVH score at 0.836 (95% CI, 0.766–0.906), and for the mICH-A and the mICH-B score at 0.816 (95% CI, 0.740–0.892) and 0.805 (95% CI,

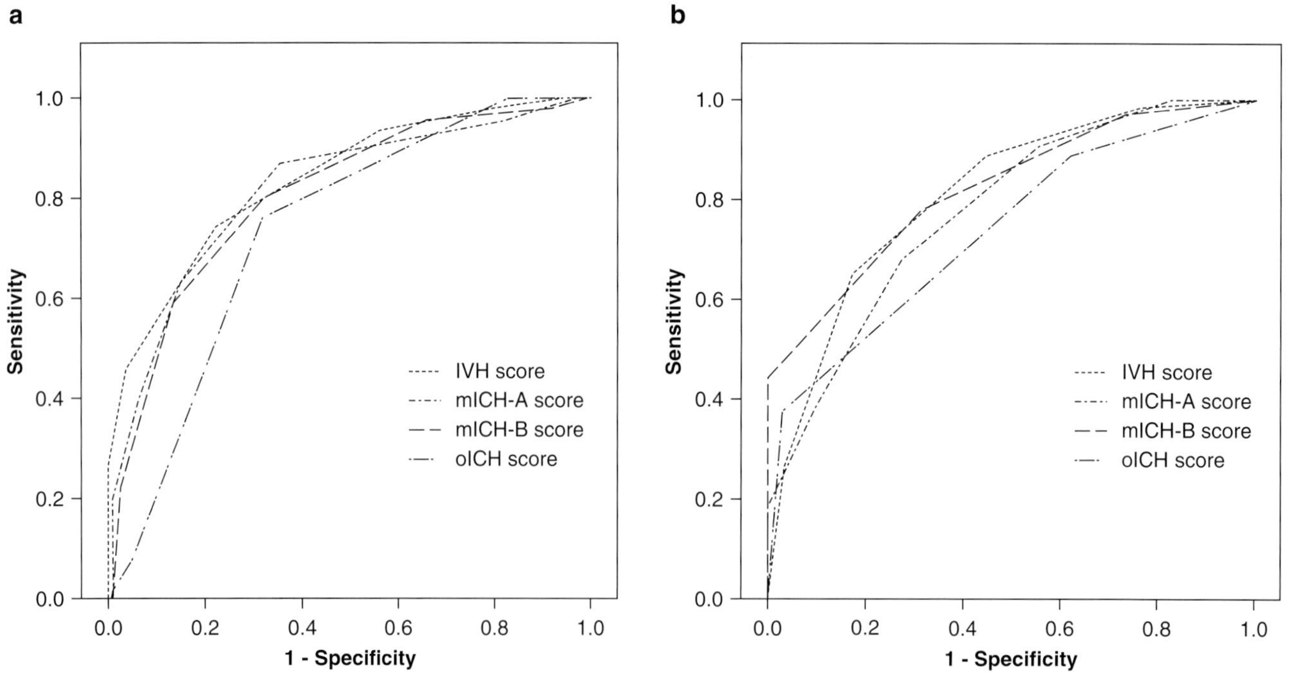

Fig. 1 ROC curve analysis with AUC for 30-day mortality (**a**) and functional outcome (**b**)

Table 1 Characteristics of 161 patients with secondary IVH

Age, years	36–86 (62.8 ± 11.2)*
GCS	3–15 (8.7 ± 3.3)*
Hematoma side *n* (%)	
Left	72 (44.7)
Right	89 (55.3)
Localization *n* (%)	
Putminal	56 (34.8)
Thalamic	62 (38.5)
Caudate	23 (14.3)
Total basal ganglia	20 (12.4)
Volume of hematoma, cm³	0.5–118.7 (27.6 ± 23.0)*
Hydrocephalus *n* (%)	93 (89.4)
Absent	13 (8.1)
Beginning	32 (19.9)
Moderate	84 (52.2)
Severe	32 (19.9)
Graeb score	2–12 (6.6 ± 2.4)*

*Mean ± SD

0.729–880). The original ICH score showed the lowest accuracy with an AUC of 0.736 (95% CI, 0.656–0.816).

In predicting the functional outcome, the highest AUC was found for the mICH-B score with an AUC of 0.823 (95% CI, 0.740–0.907). The AUCs for the IVH score and mICH-A score were 0.811 (95% CI, 0.717–0.907) and 0.778 (95% CI, 0.677–0.878), respectively. For the oICH score an AUC of 0.738 (95% CI, 0.635–0.841) was observed.

Discussion

The IVH and the mICH scores are comparable in predicting 30-day mortality. In the prediction of functional outcome, the mICH-B score followed by the IVH score reached the highest AUC. For the oICH score, only fair accuracy was calculated.

The IVH score [14] only includes components that can be identified easily during acute management in the emergency department and on the initial CT scan. The only additional score to determine is the GCS. The GCS is also part of the other tested scores.

The mICH score [7] includes the Graeb score [8] for quantifying blood in the ventricles. The mICH-A and mICH-B scores use different cut-off points for the Graeb score, GCS, and age.

The oICH score [9] contains the highest age cut-off with <80 and ≥80 years, and is the only score that includes one additional point for an infratentorial origin of hemorrhage.

The inclusion of variables like the Graeb score or hydrocephalus grading into an ICH scoring system improves the prediction of 30-day mortality and functional outcome at 6 months in SICH with secondary IVH.

Conflict of interest statement We declare that we have no conflict of interest.

References

1. Broderick J, Connolly S, Feldmann E, Hanley D et al (2007) Guidelines for the management of spontaneous intracerebral hemorrhage in adults: 2007 update: a guideline from the American Heart Association/American Stroke Association Stroke Council, High Blood Pressure Research Council, and the Quality of Care and Outcomes in Research Interdisciplinary Working Group. Circulation 116:e391–e413
2. Cheung RT, Zou LY (2003) Use of the original, modified, or new intracerebral hemorrhage score to predict mortality and morbidity after intracerebral hemorrhage. Stroke 34:1717–1722
3. Clarke JL, Johnston SC, Farrant M, Bernstein R, Tong D, Hemphill JC 3rd (2004) External validation of the ICH score. Neurocrit Care 1:53–60. doi:NCC:1:1:53 [pii]
4. Diringer MN, Edwards DF, Zazulia AR (1998) Hydrocephalus: a previously unrecognized predictor of poor outcome from supratentorial intracerebral hemorrhage. Stroke 29:1352–1357
5. Engelhard HH, Andrews CO, Slavin KV, Charbel FT (2003) Current management of intraventricular hemorrhage. Surg Neurol 60:15–21, discussion 21–12
6. Fernandes HGB, Siddique MS, Mendelow AD (2002) Testing the ICH score. Stroke 33:1455–1456
7. Godoy DA, Pinero G, Di Napoli M (2006) Predicting mortality in spontaneous intracerebral hemorrhage: can modification to original score improve the prediction? Stroke 37:1038–1044
8. Graeb DA, Robertson WD, Lapointe JS, Nugent RA, Harrison PB (1982) Computed tomographic diagnosis of intraventricular hemorrhage. Etiology and prognosis. Radiology 143:91–96
9. Hemphill JC III, Bonovich DC, Besmertis L, Manley GT, Johnston SC (2001) The ICH score: a simple, reliable grading scale for intracerebral hemorrhage. Stroke 32:891–897
10. Jamora RD, Kishi-Generao EM Jr, Bitanga ES, Gan RN, Apaga NE, San Jose MC (2003) The ICH score: predicting mortality and functional outcome in an Asian population. Stroke 34:6–7
11. Kothari RU, Brott T, Broderick JP, Barsan WG, Sauerbeck LR, Zuccarello M, Khoury J (1996) The ABCs of measuring intracerebral hemorrhage volumes. Stroke 27:1304–1305
12. Phan TG, Koh M, Vierkant RA, Wijdicks EF (2000) Hydrocephalus is a determinant of early mortality in putaminal hemorrhage. Stroke 31:2157–2162
13. Ruiz-Sandoval JL, Chiquete E, Romero-Vargas S, Padilla-Martinez JJ, Gonzalez-Cornejo S (2007) Grading scale for prediction of outcome in primary intracerebral hemorrhages. Stroke 38: 1641–1644
14. Stein M, Luecke M, Preuss M, Boeker D, Joedicke A, Oertel M (2010) Spontaneous intracerebral hemorrhage (SICH) with ventricular extension and the grading of obstructive hydrocephalus – the prediction of outcome of a special, life threatening entity. Neurosurgery 67(5):1245–1251, D-09-00922R1
15. Tuhrim S, Horowitz DR, Sacher M, Godbold JH (1995) Validation and comparison of models predicting survival following intracerebral hemorrhage. Crit Care Med 23:950–954
16. Tuhrim S, Horowitz DR, Sacher M, Godbold JH (1999) Volume of ventricular blood is an important determinant of outcome in supratentorial intracerebral hemorrhage. Crit Care Med 27:617–621

Arterial Occlusive Disease and EC-IC Bypass

Characteristics of Carotid Plaque Findings on Ultrasonography and Black Blood Magnetic Resonance Imaging in Comparison with Pathological Findings

Daisuke Arai, Susumu Yamaguchi, Mamoru Murakami, Takuya Nakakuki, Shunichi Fukuda, Noriko Satoh-Asahara, and Tetsuya Tsukahara

Abstract *Background*: Criteria to decide whether carotid endarterectomy (CEA) or carotid artery stenting (CAS) is the best mode of therapy in a specific case of cervical carotid stenosis have not been established. Overall, recent randomized clinical trials have reported that the effect on the prevention of stroke is not significantly different between CEA and CAS. CEA is more appropriate than CAS for soft atherosclerotic plaques, since such soft plaques are associated with a high incidence of ischemic complications during CAS. Therefore identification of the plaque type with noninvasive preoperative examinations plays an important role for selecting the suitable surgical method, CEA or CAS.

Objective: The objective of this study was to evaluate the association among findings of carotid ultrasonography (carotid US), black blood magnetic resonance imaging (BB-MRI), and the histopathological findings of plaque specimens removed during CEA, and secondly to consider whether these diagnostic tools are useful to predict the characteristics of carotid plaques.

Method: We investigated a total of 25 consecutive patients who underwent CEA from November 2008 to June 2010 at Kyoto Medical Center. We examined carotid plaque in 17 patients employing both carotid US and BB-MRI, 7 patients by carotid US, and 1 patient by BB-MRI. The plaque echogenicity was qualitatively assessed as low, intermediate, or high, and the MR signal intensity of the carotid plaque was classified as low or high compared with the intensity of the ipsilateral sternocleidomastoid muscle. The plaque specimens were macroscopically and pathophysiologically classified as soft or hard plaque.

Results: All low-echogenic plaques on carotid US were histologically soft plaques. The high-intensity plaques on T1-weighted imaging (T1WI) showed a tendency toward soft plaque. Thirteen of 14 plaques with high signal intensity on T1WI were morphologically soft. Eleven of 14 plaques with an intermediate echogenicity on carotid US were also morphologically soft.

Conclusion: The findings of carotid ultrasonography and BB-MRI are closely associated with the CEA specimen's morphology. Ultrasonography alone is insufficient to diagnose the plaque type accurately in some patients. Employing both carotid US and BB-MRI is useful for evaluating the characteristics of carotid plaque.

Keywords Carotid stenosis · Carotid plaque · Plaque morphology · Black blood MRI · Ultrasonography · Carotid endarterectomy

Introduction

According to a recent randomized clinical trial, outcomes of surgical treatment (CEA) and carotid artery stenting (CAS) for cervical atherosclerotic carotid artery stenosis are comparable [2, 6, 9, 13]. Therapeutic guidelines for surgical treatment have been based on the degree of stenosis and presence of neurological deficits [2], but there are still no criteria to decide on the optimal method for the individual situation, CEA or CAS.

A so-called soft plaque is vulnerable, histologically characterized by a lipid (gruel) rich core, a thin overlying fibrous cap, inflammatory infiltrate, neovasculature, and intraplaque hemorrhage. Soft plaque has a marked tendency to cause ischemic events due to cerebral emboli originating from a thrombus on the plaque surface or plaque rupture [8]. Recently, the number of patients treated with CAS has been increasing because of its lower level of invasiveness and

D. Arai (✉), S. Yamaguchi, M. Murakami, T. Nakakuki, S. Fukuda, and T. Tsukahara
Department of Neurosurgery, National Hospital Organization, Kyoto Medical Center, 1-1 Mukaihata-cho, Fukakusa, Fushimi-ku, 612-8555 Kyoto, Japan
e-mail: daisuke_arai1981@yahoo.co.jp

N. Satoh-Asahara
Division of Diabetic Research, Clinical Research Institute, National Hospital Organization, Kyoto Medical Center, Kyoto, Japan

associated shorter hospitalization time required. However, CEA is more suitable than CAS for soft plaques, which are associated with a higher incidence of ischemic complications during CAS [1, 4, 7]. It is important to understand these plaque characteristics in order to choose the most appropriate treatment method.

Carotid ultrasonography (US) has been widely applied to evaluate plaque morphology. However, carotid US has some limitations in the presence of a short neck, high carotid bifurcation, or back shadow due to plaque calcification. Furthermore, image interpretation is influenced by the subjective evaluation of the examiner.

Recent studies have reported on the feasibility of black blood magnetic resonance imaging (BB-MRI) as an accurate tool for identifying carotid plaque characteristics. In addition to this, BB-MRI can identify plaque components, such as gruel, intraplaque hemorrhage, and fibrous tissue on the basis of the MR signal intensity [5, 10, 11, 12, 14]. Thus, the combination of US and BB-MRI can be useful as a noninvasive method for detecting the plaque type.

To our knowledge, however, few studies have evaluated the association between the noninvasive identifications of the plaque type and histopathological findings. Here, we evaluated the usefulness of carotid US and BB-MRI as preoperative diagnostic tools for identifying carotid plaque characteristics compared to histopathological findings of specimens obtained during CEA.

Methods

A total of 25 consecutive patients who had undergone CEA from November 2008 to June 2010 in the National Hospital Organization Kyoto Medical Center were recruited for this study after having given informed consent. We preoperatively examined the carotid plaque characteristics using carotid US and/or BB-MRI: 17 patients underwent both carotid US and BB-MRI, 7 patients carotid US only, and 1 patient BB-MRI only.

Carotid Ultrasonography

The carotid arteries were examined bilaterally at the levels of the common carotid artery, carotid bifurcation, and internal carotid arteries from transverse and longitudinal orientations. Gain setting and continuous angle adjustment were used to optimize image quality. Carotid plaque was defined as an arterial wall lesion that projected into the vessel lumen. The plaque echogenicity was qualitatively assessed as being on average low (blood-like echogenicity), intermediate, or high (intensely bright echogenicity).

Black Blood MRI

We performed carotid artery BB-MRI using a 1.5-T Philips imaging machine with a protocol that generated two contrast weightings (T1-weighted image and T2-weighted image). MRI was conducted using cardiac gating to minimize the motion artifact and the fat suppression method to suppress marked signal hyperintensity due to subcutaneous fat tissue. We obtained T1- and T2-weighted short axis images of the artery, including the area with the highest degree of stenosis. The MR signal intensity of the carotid plaque in the area with the highest rate of stenosis was classified as low or high compared with the intensity of the ipsilateral sternocleidomastoid muscle.

Plaque Specimens

The plaque specimens obtained during CEA were excised en bloc, and an incision was made in all 25 specimens to analyze the type of plaque. The plaque specimens were macroscopically classified as soft or hard. We defined gruel or intraplaque hemorrhage as soft, and fibrosity or calcification as hard.

Results

As shown in Fig. 1a, low-intensity plaques on T1WI and T2WI were all defined as hard on histological examination, and 13 of 14 plaques showing high signal intensity on T1WI were morphologically soft.

All low-echogenic plaques were histologically soft, and 4 of 5 high-echoic plaques were histologically hard (Fig. 1b). One high-echogenic plaque with poor image quality due to the presence of a back shadow was histologically soft. Of 14 plaques evaluated as intermediate on carotid US examination, 11 were histologically soft, and three were hard.

The diagnostic rate of soft plaque was 79% on carotid US and 93% on BB-MRI. When the carotid US findings of plaque showed intermediate echogenicity, employing BB-MRI helped in the accurate evaluation of the plaque type. As shown in Fig. 1c, the majority of high-intensity plaques on T1WI among plaques with intermediate echogenicity were histologically soft.

Figure 2 shows US and MRI images and the pathology in a typical case with soft plaque.

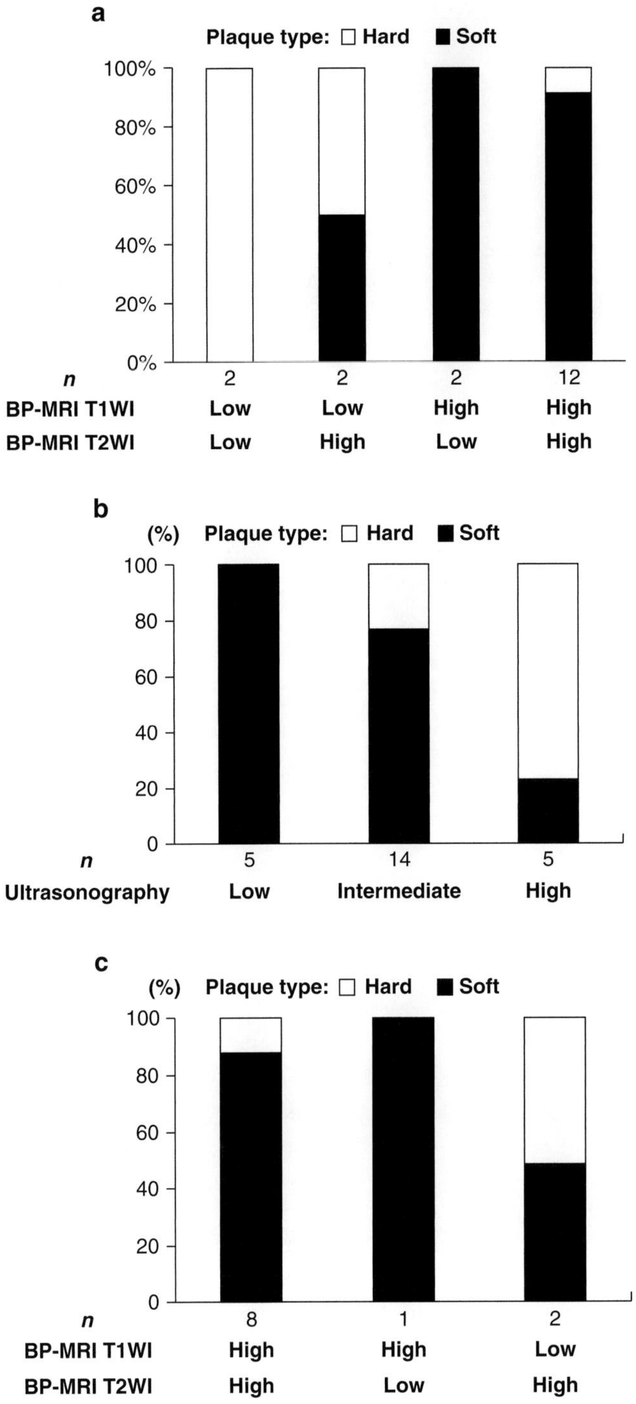

Fig. 1 Comparison of the characteristics of atherosclerotic carotid plaque based on the preoperative examination and histological findings. (**a**) Comparison of black blood MRI and histological findings ($n = 18$). *Black box* shows the rate of soft plaque on each MRI finding. (**b**) Comparison of ultasound characteristics and histological findings ($n = 24$). *Black box* shows the rate of soft plaque on each ultrasonographic finding. (**c**) Comparison between black blood MRI and histological findings of those plaques with intermediate ultrasound characteristics ($n = 11$). *Black box* shows the rate of soft plaque on each MRI finding

Discussion

As a general rule, echolucent plaques on carotid US are soft, whereas echogenic plaques are hard because of the higher content of fibrous tissue and calcification. Our results were consistent with this assumption. However, in one patient we could not accurately diagnose the character of the plaque because of a back shadow. Poor plaque imaging on carotid US may hamper an accurate diagnosis. If the plaque showed an intermediate echogenicity on carotid US, about 30% were histologically hard. Intermediate echogenicity can be influenced by the subjective evaluation of the examiner. This is a limitation of qualitative evaluation on carotid US.

BB-MRI has been considered useful in diagnosing the chemical composition and physical properties of tissue in the carotid artery. It is possible to evaluate the characteristics of carotid plaques objectively using the MR signal intensity. T1-weighted MR sequences are commonly used to detect intraplaque hemorrhage, which results in T1 shortening and correspondingly causes high signal intensity on T1-weighted MR images. Intraplaque hemorrhage in the atherosclerotic lesions is thought to be a critical entity in the progression of atherosclerosis because of the deposition of free cholesterol, macrophage infiltration, and enlargement of the necrotic core caused by the accumulation of erythrocyte membranes within an atherosclerotic plaque. Therefore, intraplaque hemorrhage is a risk of plaque destabilization [5]. Recent studies have reported that high intensity on T1WI reliably indicates soft plaque [10, 11, 12, 14].

In our investigation, on T1WI high-intensity plaques showed a tendency to be histologically soft. The diagnostic accuracy for detecting soft plaque on BB-MRI was higher than on carotid US.

Carotid artery stenosis is an important cause of stroke and may cause 10–20% of all cases of ischemic stroke. Large randomized controlled trials have demonstrated the effect of both CEA and CAS on stroke prevention in patients with carotid stenosis [2, 3, 6, 9, 13]. However, in the presence of soft plaque, CEA is recommended. Therefore, the preoperative evaluation of carotid plaque morphology is important.

Here we show that carotid US and BB-MRI findings correlated with the histopathological findings, but there were cases in which US alone was insufficient to diagnose the plaque type accurately. In such cases, examination with BB-MRI in addition to US was useful. We think that carotid US and BB-MRI are valuable diagnostic tools to help choose between the treatment methods of CEA or CAS.

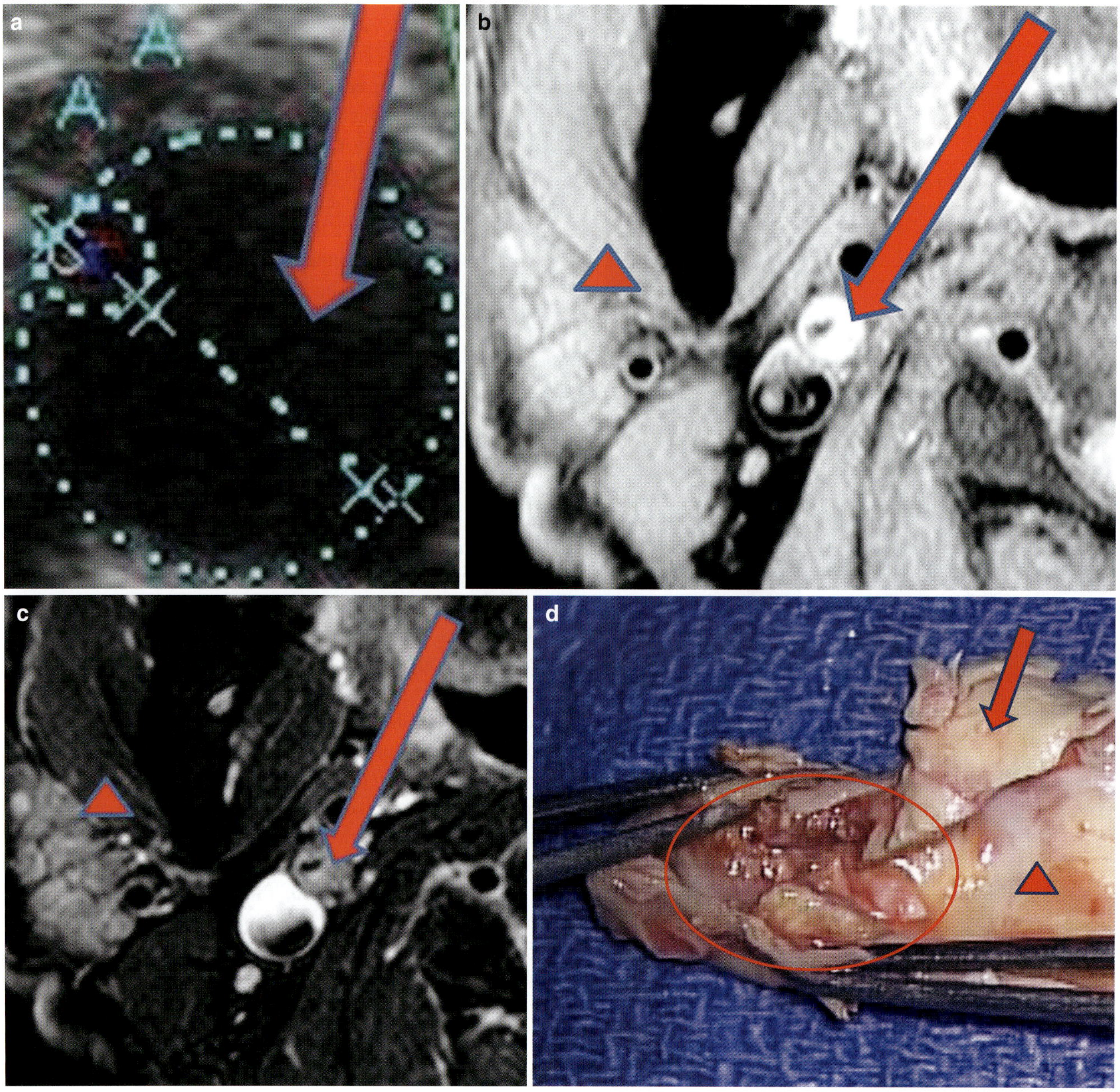

Fig. 2 US, MRI, and histological images of a typical soft plaque. (**a**) Ultrasonographic short axis image of carotid plaque. The *red arrow* shows low echoic plaque at the origin of the right internal carotid artery. (**b**) Axial T1-weighted image of the origin of the right internal carotid artery. The *red arrow* shows high-intensity plaque. *Red arrowhead* shows the right sternocleidomastoid muscle. (**c**) Axial T2-weighted image of the origin of the right internal carotid artery. The *red arrow* shows high-intensity plaque. *Red arrowhead* shows the right sternocleidomastoid muscle. (**d**) Macroscopic image of a specimen incised during CEA. *Red circle* shows soft plaque, *red arrow* shows the right external carotid artery, and the *red arrowhead* shows the right common carotid artery. (**e**) Histopathological finding of carotid plaque obtained during CEA (Elastica van Gieson stain, ×40) indicates a lipid core (*red circle*). *Red arrowhead* shows true lumen

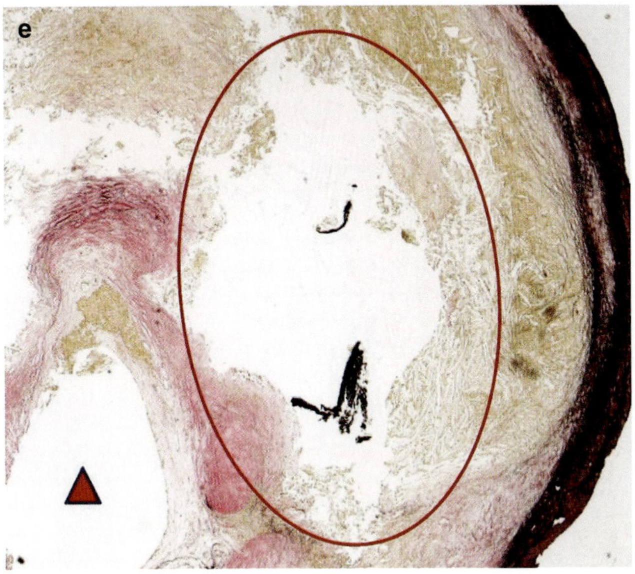

Fig. 2 (continued)

Conflict of interest statement We declare that we have no conflict of interest.

References

1. Biasi GM, Froio A (2004) Carotid plaque echolucency increases the risk of stroke in carotid stenting: the Imaging in Carotid Angioplasty and Risk of Stroke (ICAROS) study. Circulation 110:756–762
2. Ederle J, Dobson J (2010) Carotid artery stenting compared with endarterectomy in patients with symptomatic carotid stenosis (International Carotid Stenting Study): an interim analysis of a randomized controlled trial. Lancet 375:985–997
3. Halliday A, Mansfield A (2004) Prevention of disabling and fatal strokes by successful carotid endarterectomy in patients without recent neurological symptoms: randomized controlled trial. Lancet 363:1491–1502
4. Henry M, Henry I (2002) Benefits of cerebral protection during carotid stenting with the PercuSurge GuardWire system: midterm results. J Endovasc Ther 9:1–13
5. Kolodgie FD, Gold HK (2003) Intraplaque hemorrhage and progression of coronary atheroma. N Engl J Med 349:2316–2325
6. Mas JL, Chatellier G (2006) Endarterectomy versus stenting in patients with symptomatic severe carotid stenosis. N Engl J Med 355:1660–1671
7. Ohki T, Marin ML (1998) Ex vivo human carotid artery bifurcation stenting: correlation of lesion characteristics with embolic potential. J Vasc Surg 27:463–471
8. Redgrave JN, Lovett JK et al (2006) Histological assessment of 526 symptomatic carotid plaques in relation to the nature and timing of ischemic symptoms: Oxford plaque study. Circulation 113: 2320–2328
9. Ringleb PA, Allenberg J (2006) 30 day results from the SPACE trial of stent-protected angioplasty versus carotid endarterectomy in symptomatic patients: a randomized non-inferiority trial. Lancet 36:1239–1247
10. Rothwell PM, Eliasziw M (2004) Endarterectomy for symptomatic carotid stenosis in relation to clinical subgroups and timing of surgery. Lancet 363:915–924
11. Saam T, Hatsukami TS (2007) The vulnerable, or high-risk, atherosclerotic plaque: noninvasive MR imaging for characterization and assessment. Radiology 244:64–77
12. Touze E, Toussaint JF (2007) Reproducibility of high-resolution MRI for the identification and the quantification of carotid atherosclerotic plaque components: consequences for prognosis studies and therapeutic trials. Stroke 38:1812–1819
13. Yadav JS, Wholey MH (2004) Protected carotid-artery stenting versus endarterectomy in high-risk patients. N Engl J Med 351:1493–1501
14. Yoshida K (2008) Characterization of carotid atherosclerosis and detection of soft plaque with use of black-blood MR imaging. Am J Neuroradiol 29:868–874

Indication for Surgical Treatment of Carotid Arterial Stenosis in High-Risk Patients

Tetsuya Tsukahara, Shunichi Fukuda, Takuya Nakakuki, Mamoru Murakami, Daisuke Arai, and Susumu Yamaguchi

Abstract The indication for carotid endarterectomy (CEA) or carotid artery stenting (CAS) has not been established, although the beneficial effects of these surgical treatments for severe cervical carotid stenosis have been confirmed by clinical trial studies. We report our clinical results of CAS and CEA and suggest an appropriate treatment strategy, especially for high-risk patients. From January 2001 to December 2009, we treated 171 carotid lesions by CEA and 251 lesions by CAS. Stenosis was symptomatic in 68%, and the average stenotic rate was 83% in the CEA group. In the CAS group, stenosis was symptomatic in 62%, and the average stenotic rate was 65%. Stenosis was relieved in all cases after CEA or CAS. Surgical mortality with CEA and CAS was 0.6% (1/171) and 0.4% (1/251), respectively. Surgical morbidity by ischemic stroke with CEA and CAS was 2.9% (5/171) and 1.2% (3/251), respectively. Surgical morbidity was not increased in patients with medical risk factors. The long-term outcome after CAS was not inferior to that after CEA. In conclusion, carotid stenosis can be treated with comparably low morbidity and mortality rates using CEA or CAS even in high-risk patients when the method is appropriately selected considering the characteristics of the carotid stenosis.

Keywords Carotid endarterectomy (CEA) · Carotid artery stenting (CAS)

Introduction

The benefit of surgical intervention for severe carotid stenosis has been confirmed by randomized clinical trials (RCT) [2, 4]. Two surgical therapeutic methods are available, carotid endarterectomy (CEA) and carotid artery stenting (CAS), although no indication for CEA or CAS for cervical carotid stenosis has been established yet. A recent RCT reported that the stroke prevention effect was not statistically different between CEA and CAS for CEA high-risk patients [6]; however, to achieve a better outcome with surgical treatments, we have to select CEA or CAS considering not only the patient's condition, but also the characteristics of carotid stenosis and plaque.

In this study, we report our clinical therapeutic results of CAS and CEA and suggest an appropriate treatment strategy, especially for high-risks patient.

Materials and Methods

From January 2001 to December 2009, we treated cervical carotid stenosis surgically in 171 lesions by CEA and 251 lesions by CAS. CEA was considered the first choice of the surgical treatment for severe carotid stenosis, especially with soft plaque, eccentric or tortuous lesions, and a narrow residual lumen with massive carotid plaque. CAS was chosen when CEA was considered to be high risk with: (1) a contralateral ICA lesion, (2) distal carotid lesion, (3) higher cervical lesion and (4) medical risk factors, such as untreated coronary heart disease. For bilateral carotid lesions, the milder carotid stenosis was first treated by CAS, and then the more severe stenosis was treated by CEA. The average patient age was 69.5 in the CEA group and 71.0 for CAS. The stenosis was symptomatic in 68% of the CEA patients, and the average stenotic rate was 83%. For CAS, stenosis was symptomatic in 62% and the average stenotic rate was 65% (Table 1). Medical risk factors of both groups are shown in Table 1. Short-term surgical results were examined by follow-up MRA, MRI, 3DCTA or DSA angiography. Long-term results were also examined in 352 carotid stenotic lesions treated before May 2007.

T. Tsukahara (✉), S. Fukuda, T. Nakakuki, M. Murakami, D. Arai, and S. Yamaguchi
Department of Neurosurgery, National Hospital Organization, Kyoto Medical Center, 1-1 Mukaihata-cho, Fukakusa, Fushimi-ku, 612–8555 Kyoto, Japan
e-mail: ttsukaha@kyotolan.hosp.go.jp

T. Tsukahara et al. (eds.), *Trends in Neurovascular Surgery*, Acta Neurochirurgica Supplementum, Vol. 112,
DOI: 10.1007/978-3-7091-0661-7_4, © Springer-Verlag/Wien 2011

Table 1 Characteristics of patients and carotid stenosis, and medical risk factors

	Age (mean)	Male	HT	DM	HL	CHD/ untreated (%)	Symptomatic (%)	Stenosis (%)
CEA	69.5	82	70	24	20	19/0	68	83
CAS	71.0	80	40	18	21	10/5	62	65

HT hypertension, *DM* diabetes mellitus, *HL* hyperlipidemia, *CHD* coronary heart disease

Results

Short-Term Results

The surgical results are summarized in Table 2. Stenosis of the carotid arteries was relieved in all cases after CEA as well as CAS. Surgical mortality with CEA and CAS was 0.6% (1/171) and 0.4% (1/251), respectively. Surgical morbidity with ischemic stroke was 2.9% (5/171) for CEA and 2.4% (6/251) for CAS, respectively. One patient with untreated coronary heart disease suffered acute myocardial infarction after CAS. Surgical morbidity was not significantly elevated in patients with medical risk factors.

Long-Term Results

The average follow-up period was 31.2 months after CEA and CAS. Mortality was 8.2% after CEA, and 5.0% after CAS, and mRS (modified Rankin Scale) scores of the patients decreased by 0.33 after CEA and by 0.48 after CAS, respectively, during the follow-up period.

Table 2 Surgical results

CEA			
Death (renal failure, MOF)	1	0.75%	(1/134)
Major stroke	1	0.75%	(1/134)
Minor stroke	3	2.24%	(3/134)
Restenosis	9	6.71%	(9/134)
CAS			
Death (blue toe syndrome, MOF)	1	0.46%	(1/218)
Major stroke	3	1.38%	(3/218)
Minor stroke	1	0.46%	(1/218)
Restenosis	6	2.75%	(6/218)

Case Presentations: Complications After Surgical Treatment

Case 1: An 84-year-old woman with diabetes, hypertension and hyperlipidemia came to our clinic for surgery of asymptomatic carotid stenosis. The preoperative studies revealed a 90% stenosis of the left ICA and an 80% stenosis of the right ICA. Right carotid stenosis was first treated by CAS (Fig. 1), and left carotid stenosis was treated by CEA 3 days after CAS (Fig. 2a). After left CEA, she had right hemiparesis due to infarction of the left basal ganglia and corona radiata (Fig. 2b).

Case 2: A 74-year-old man with hypertension and renal failure suffered from weakness of the right lower limb. Angiography revealed an 80% stenosis of the left ICA and 70% stenosis of the right ICA. Four days after successful CAS of the left ICA, he suffered from ileus caused by embolic occlusion of the superior mesencepharic artery (Fig. 3a, b).

Discussion

The *Stenting and Angioplasty with Protection in Patients at High Risk for Endarterectomy* (SAPPHIRE) trial was the first completed controlled, prospective randomized trial in which CEA was compared with state of the art CAS with cerebral protection [6]. The SAPPHIRE trial only enrolled patients who were considered at high risk for CEA, i.e., octogenarians and those with carotid reoperation, cervical radiation, contralateral carotid occlusion, severe tandem lesions, high cervical lesions (at least C2), lesions below the clavicle, and contralateral laryngeal palsy. The perioperative risks of stroke (CAS, 3.1%, CEA, 3.3%) and mortality (CAS 0.6%, CEA 2.0%) were similar; however, more patients suffered postoperative myocardial infarction (MI) in the CEA group than in the CAS group. In our series of treatments we chose CAS for patients with untreated coronary disease. After the coronary disease had been treated and was stable, CEA did not induce MI in the perioperative period. A recent international randomized controlled trial (RCT) comparing CAS with CEA in patients with symptomatic carotid stenosis

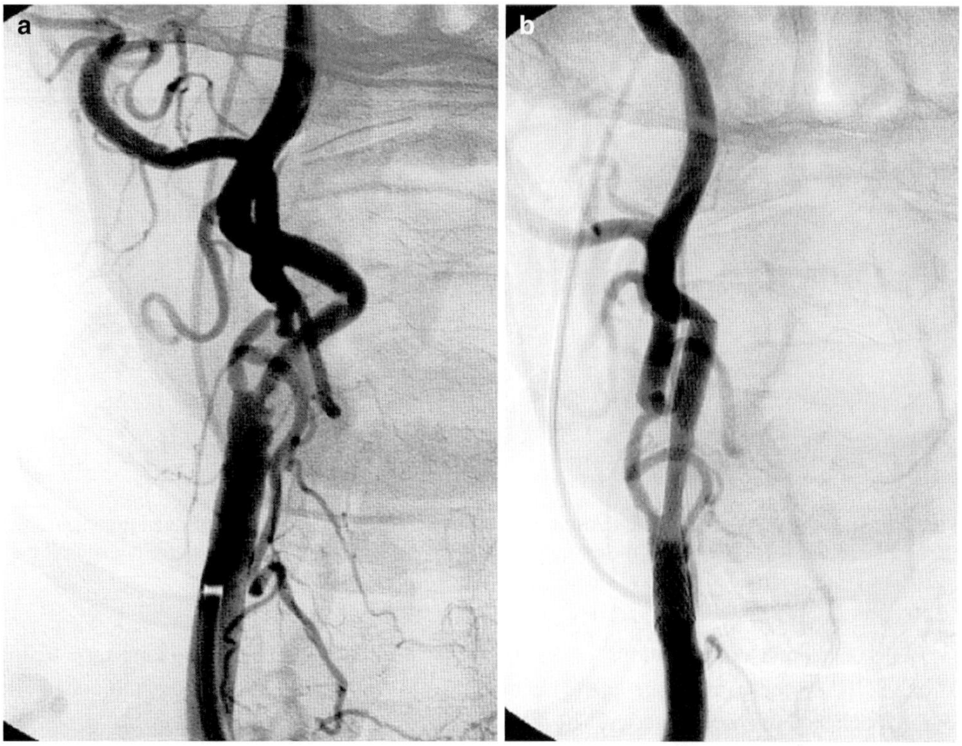

Fig. 1 Case 1: Preoperative angiography revealed 80% stenosis of the right ICA (**a**). Right carotid stenosis was first treated by CAS (**b**)

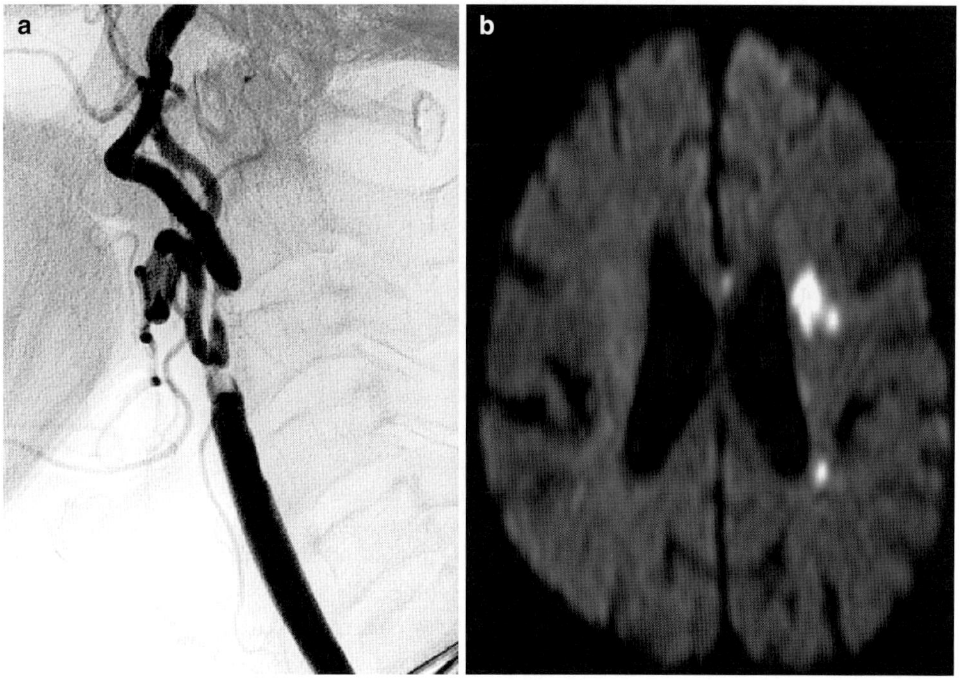

Fig. 2 Left carotid stenosis was treated by CEA 3 days after CAS (**a**). After left CEA, the patient had right hemiparesis due to infarction of the left basal ganglia and corona radiata (**b**)

reported that the incidence of stroke, death or procedural myocardial infarction was 8.5% in the CAS group compared with 5.2% in the CEA group [3]. The risks of any stroke and all-cause death were higher in the CAS group than in the CEA group. Another recent international RCT also reported the superior stroke prevention effect of CEA over CAS [1]. In our series of treatments, when compared with the results of RCTs, CEA and CAS for carotid stenosis were performed with a comparably low rate of complications even in high-risk patients. These results suggest that our treatment strategy for carotid stenosis is basically acceptable, although there are some points for discussion.

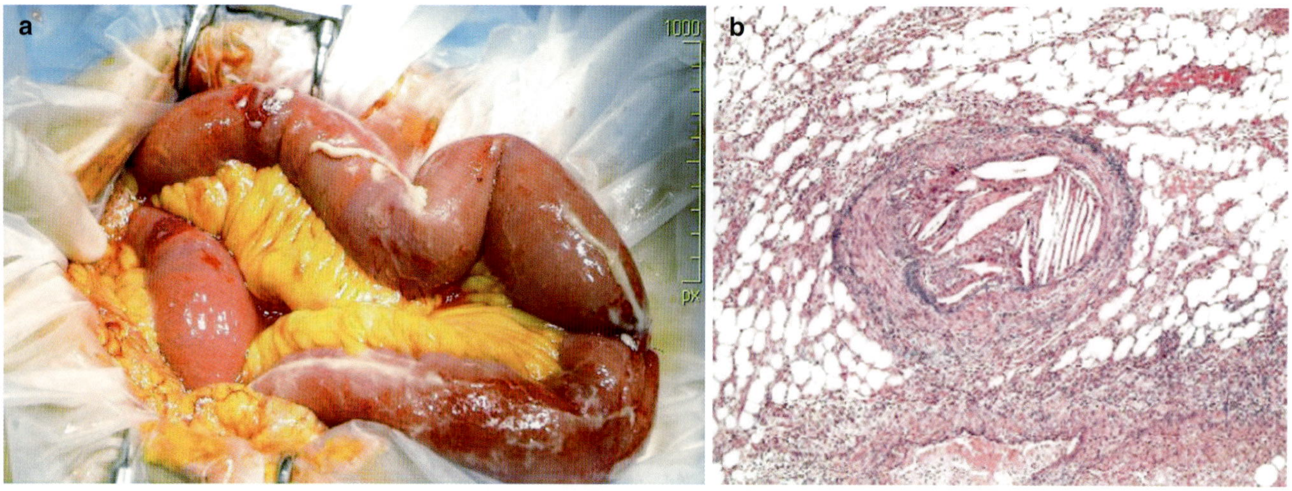

Fig. 3 Case 2: 4 days after successful CAS for left ICA stenosis, a 74-year-old man suffered from ileus. Laparotomy revealed a necrotic lesion of the small intestine (**a**). The superior mesencepharic artery of the lesion was occluded by the embolus of the cholesterin crystal (**b**)

Major ischemic complications of CEA are (1) embolic stroke in the perioperative stage and (2) hemodynamic stroke during occlusion of carotid arteries. The most important factor to prevent embolic stroke may be the surgical CEA procedure. Although it is necessary to detect the precise dissecting layer and not to leave a piece of plaque at the distal end of the ICA, this procedure is sometimes complicated and is not easy, especially when the lesion is located at a high cervical level [5]. In case 1, we performed CEA without using an internal shunt after increasing crossflow by contralateral CAS. Crossflow may not be sufficient during closure of the ICA. We used an internal shunt for selective cases to prevent hemodynamic stroke. Since it sometimes increases the risk of embolic stroke to insert a shunt in a distal ICA region, an internal shunt should be used for selective cases after examining cerebral blood flow after cross clamping the carotid arteries.

A major complication of CAS is embolic stroke due to dilatation of the stenotic lesion and plaque. Since the recent development of MRI and Doppler echography has enabled us to detect the characteristics of the carotid plaque, we should select CAS or CEA according to the plaque morphology. Another major complication of CAS is apparently embolism during catheterization of eccentric and tortuous sclerotic arteries. As shown in case 2, embolic complications can occur not only in the brain, but also in other peripheral arteries. We also experienced mortality as a result of complications of catheterization, such as blue toe syndrome. We should therefore select CEA for severe carotid stenosis and tortuous lesions after studying the aortic arteries by 3DCTA or DSA angiography.

In conclusion, carotid stenotic lesions can be treated with comparably low morbidity and mortality rates using CEA and CAS even in patients with medical comorbidity or bilateral carotid stenosis. CAS is not inferior to CEA with regard to the long-term results. The most appropriate method should be selected considering the individual characteristics of carotid stenosis.

Conflict of interest statement We declare that we have no conflict of interest.

References

1. Brott TG, Hobson RW, Howard G, Roubin GS, Clark WM, Brooks W, Mackey A, Hill MD, Leimgruber PP, Sheffet AJ, Howard VJ, Moore WS, Voeks JH, Hopkins LN, Cutlip DE, Cohen DJ, Popma JJ, Ferguson RD, Cohen SN, Blackshear JL, Silver FL, Mohr JP, Lal BK, Meschia JF, for the CREST Investigators (2010) Stenting versus endarterectomy for treatment of carotid-artery stenosis. N Engl J Med 363:11–23
2. CAVATAS investigators (2001) Endovascular versus surgical treatment in patients with carotid stenosis in the Carotid and Vertebral Artery Transluminal Angioplasty Study (CAVATAS): a randomised trial. Lancet 357:1729–1737
3. International Carotid Stenting Study Investigators (2010) Carotid artery stenting compared with endarterectomy in patients with symptomatic carotid stenosis (International Carotid Stenting Study): an interim analysis of a randomised controlled trial. Lancet 375:985–997
4. North American Symptomatic Carotid Endarterectomy Trial Collaborators (1991) Beneficial effect of carotid endarterectomy in symptomatic patients with high-grade carotid stenosis. N Engl J Med 325:445–453
5. Tsukahara T, Akiyama Y, Nomura MMD, Hashimoto NMD (1977) Carotid endarterectomy: standard techniques to avoid complications. Jpn J Neurosurg 6(11):731–736
6. Yadav JS, Wholey MH, Kuntz RE, Fayad P, Katzen BT, Gj M, Bajwa TK, Whitlow P, Strickman NE, Jaff MR, Popma JJ, Snead DB, Cutlip DE, Firth BG, Ouriel K (2004) Protected carotid-artery stenting versus endarterectomy in high-risk patients. N Engl J Med 351:1493–1501

The Impact of Early Perfusion CT Measurement After Extracranial-Intracranial Bypass Surgery: Results of a Pilot Study

Sven O. Eicker, Kerim Beseoglu, Nima Etminan, Bernd Turowski, Hans-Jakob Steiger, and Daniel Hänggi

Abstract *Objective*: The early postoperative period after extracranial-intracranial bypass surgery carries the risk of hypo- as well as hyperperfusion. The purpose of this study is to evaluate early perfusion computerized tomography (PCT) after revascularization to assess the hemodynamic balance.

Methods: Standard cerebral bypass surgery was performed on ten patients, and PCT measurement within 6 h after surgery was performed and analyzed.

Results: The hemisphere with reduced cerebral vascular reserve (CVR) showed a regional cerebral baseline blood flow (CBF) of 5.58 ± 1.69 and a regional cerebral baseline blood volume (CBV) of 2.41 ± 0.76 before surgery. Mean transit time (MTT) was 4.16 ± 0.9 s and time to peak (TTP) 3.25 ± 1.62 s. After the procedure values changed significantly ($p < 0.05$) in eight patients who had no complications. Patency rate was documented in all patients by angiography. One patient showed a decrease of CBF and CBV and an increase of MTT and TTP. Clinically the patient developed a transient hemiparesis immediately after surgery. Another patient showed the expected increase in CBF and CBV; however, MTT and TTP also increased. A delayed hemiparesis probably related to hyperperfusion occurred with improvement in the follow-up.

Conclusion: This pilot study demonstrates that early PCT parameters can provide immediate and detailed information about hemodynamic parameters and seems to have a predictive value regarding the morbidity of hypo- or hyperperfusion in patients after cerebral bypass surgery.

Keywords Early CT perfusion · Extracranial-intracranial bypass · Hyperperfusion · Hypoperfusion

S.O. Eicker (✉), K. Beseoglu, N. Etminan, B. Turowski, H.-J. Steiger, and D. Hänggi
Department of Neurosurgery, Heinrich Heine University, Moorenstraße 5, 40225 Düsseldorf, Germany
e-mail: eicker.s@mac.com

Introduction

Patients suffering from internal carotid artery (ICA) occlusive disease show a remarkable but individually variable risk of subsequent stroke. Besides clinical symptoms the impairment of the cerebral vascular reserve capacity (CVR) has been identified as the major predictive indicator for the risk of cerebral infarction [19]. Standard superficial temporal artery to middle cerebral artery (STA-MCA) bypass surgery is one treatment option for patients suffering from hemodynamically relevant ICA occlusion [13]. Intraoperative bypass patency can be evaluated using near-infrared indocyanine green (ICG) fluorescence angiography [18], microvascular Doppler and ultrasonic perivascular flow probe devices. Postoperative catheter (DSA)- or magnetic resonance (MR)-based angiography are typically used to assess bypass patency. For evaluation of the cerebral perfusion, diverse imaging modalities are available, including perfusion magnetic resonance imaging (MRI) [5], single photon emission computed tomography (SPECT) [10], positron emission tomography (PET) [2], xenon computed tomography (CT) [6], perfusion computerized tomography (PCT) [6] as well as local, invasive tools like regional cerebral blood flow [11, 15], laser Doppler flowmeter [7] or brain-tissue oxygenation measurements [9]. This multitude of modalities has different advantages and disadvantages. Except for the local procedures, most modalities are established in the following days or month after revascularization in order to identify improvements after bypass surgery. Nevertheless, perfusion changes can occur in the early postoperative period, with the risk of hypo- as well as hyperperfusion associated with severe morbidity.

The purpose of this study is to evaluate early PCT after revascularization to access the predictive hemodynamic balance in the immediate postoperative stage.

DOI: 10.1007/978-3-7091-0661-7_5,

Materials and Methods

Patient Population

Ten patients who presented in the clinic from October 2009 to March 2010 were included in this study. They suffered from symptomatic ICA occlusion or Moyamoya disease with impaired CVR and were considered for cerebral revascularization. During surgery bypass patency was evaluated by the use of ICG fluorescence angiography, microvascular Doppler and ultrasonic perivascular flow probe devices. Postoperatively all patients underwent an early PCT and the DSA. Criteria for exclusion were age under 18 years. All patients had given informed consent.

PCT Protocol

PCT was performed using a multislice CT Scanner (Volume Zoom, Siemens Erlangen/Germany, 80.0 kV, 120m As, 1 scan/s, overall duration 35 s). Patients were examined before and after acetazolamide treatment (Diamox®, 1,000 mg i.e., over 2 min) the same day preoperatively and without acetazolamide within 6 h immediately after bypass surgery. For all examinations, patients received a single bolus of 30 mL contrast agent intravenously (400 mg iodine/mL), equaling a total iodine dose of 12 g. Two 10-mm-thick slices representing all three supratentorial vascular territories were obtained. Raw data were transferred to a workstation for further processing. Analysis comprising determination of mean transit time (MTT), regional cerebral blood flow (CBF), regional cerebral blood volume (CBV) and time to peak (TTP) was carried out by STROKETOOL-CT software (version 2.0) [17]. Perfusion maps were further evaluated using the computer software Angiotux CT 2D [14]. For each hemisphere the mean values of all four perfusion parameters in 18 overlapping defined cortical segments (sections of 10° and intersections of 2°) were determined. All segments were related to vascular territories: A 40° occipital segment corresponds to the vascular territory of the posterior cerebral artery; the following 110° segment to the vascular territory of the middle cerebral artery; and the remaining 30° segment to the vascular territory of the anterior cerebral artery (Fig. 1).

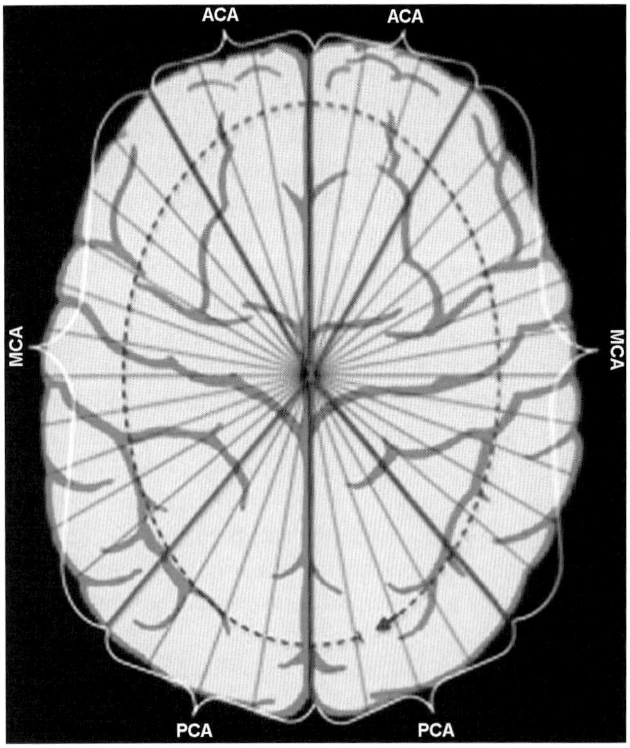

Fig. 1 Brain map divided into 36 segments to analyze the holo-hemispheric perfusion and specific vascular territories of the 110° expanded MCA territory

Results

Patient Population

Six male and four female patients with a mean age of 53.3 years (range 18–69 years) were included in the evaluation. Symptomatic unilateral ICA occlusion was present in seven patients (three right sided and four left sided) and Moyamoya disease in three. Ten EC-IC bypass surgeries were performed (STA-MCA anastomosis). A total of 20 PCT examinations were performed and compared.

Intra- and Postoperative Assessment of Bypass Patency

Intraoperative ICG fluorescence angiography confirmed the patency of the STA-MCA bypass and showed an anastomosis without obstructions in all ten patients. Intraoperative ultrasonic perivascular flow measurement demonstrated flow rates between 18 and 55 mL/min. Postoperative DSA performed 24 h after surgery showed patency in all patients.

Clinical Outcome

Eight patients had an inconspicuous follow-up in the intensive care unit (ICU) after the STA-MCA anastomotic procedure, notably without new neurological symptoms. One patient experienced a delayed (day 2 after surgery) transient hemiparesis with improvement in the follow-up (patient 1). Immediately postoperatively, another patient developed a new transient neurological deficit in terms of hemiparesis (patient 10) with good recovery.

Postoperative Changes in PCT Parameters

As expected, the average holo-hemispheric PCT values of the eight inconspicuous patients changed significantly from before to after the STA-MCA anastomosis on the hemisphere with reduced CVR. CBF increased from a baseline of 5.58 (±1.69) to 7.29 (±2.51). CBV changed from 2.41 (±0.76) to 2.57 (±0.77). A decrease in MTT and TTP confirmed the hypothesis of flow improvement. MTT altered from 4.16 s (±0.9 s) before bypass to 3.99 s (±1.11 s) after the procedure. TTP values changed from 3.25 s (±1.62 s) to 2.57 s (±1.44 s). Alterations of all four PCT parameters after bypass surgery were significant ($p<0.05$). Patient 1 showed the expected increase in CBF (5.71–6.03) and CBV (2.92–3.30), and MTT (5.43–5.84 s) and TTP (5.85–6.10 s) also increased. This patient presented with a delayed hemiparesis after hours with improvement in the follow-up. Patient 10 developed a permanent hemiparesis immediately after surgery. In this patient all four holo-hemispheric PCT parameters changed unexpectedly (CBF from 4.65 to 3.79; CBV from 2.70 to 2.0 and MTT from 3.87 to 4.2 s; TTP from 3.44 to 3.7 s) (Fig. 2). In the two patients with postoperative clinical aggravation and unexpected changes in two, respectively four PCT parameters, specific analyses of the territory of the middle cerebral artery (MCA) in the symptomatic hemisphere were performed. Perfusion parameters of this unique 110° territory presented different changes in comparison with the holo-hemispheric results. In patient 1, CBF changed from 5.76 to 4.01, CBV from 3.24 to 2.81, MTT from 5.80 to 7.12 s and TTP from 5.82 to 8.01 s. Regarding only the MCA territory, four unexpected changes were detected. In the holo-hemispheric results, patient 10 demonstrated unexpected changes in four parameters. Taking a closer look at the MCA territory, CBF increased from 3.25 to 4.50, CBV from 4.79 to 9.69, MTT from 4.80 s to 6.31 s and TTP from 4.80 s to 6.31 s. In this territory an expected but considerable increase in CBF and CBV was found. MTT and TTP also showed unexpected changes (Fig. 3).

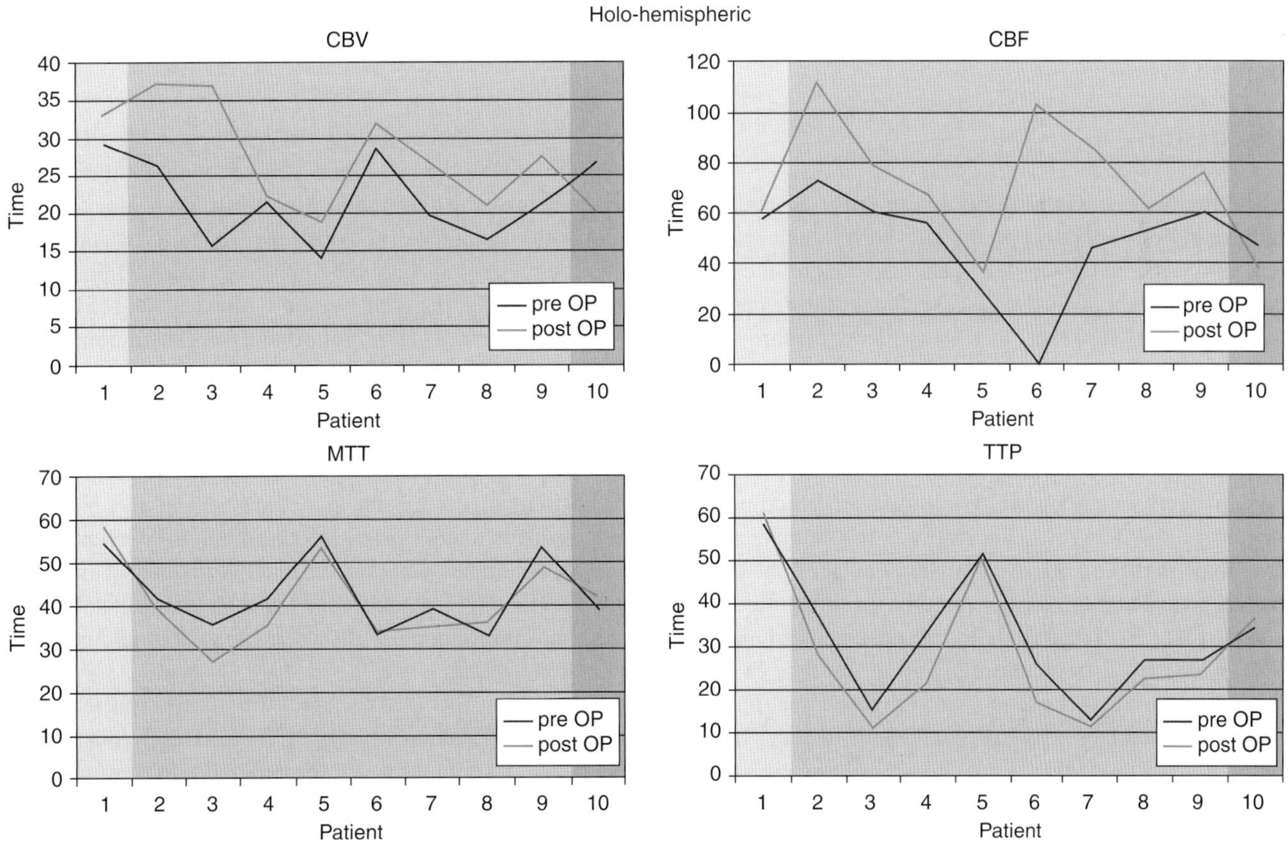

Fig. 2 Pre- and postoperative holo-hemispheric results of the CBV, CBF, MTT and TTP measurements

MCA territory

Pat 1

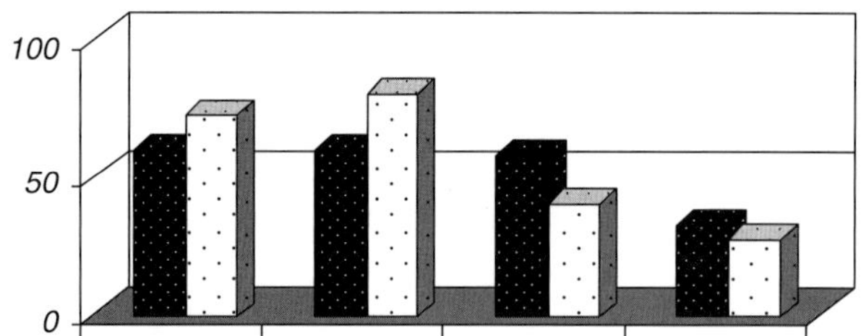

	MTT	TTP	CBF	CBV
■ Pre OP	58,001	58,166	57,64	32,46
□ Post OP	71,97	80,49	40,08	28,07

Pat 10

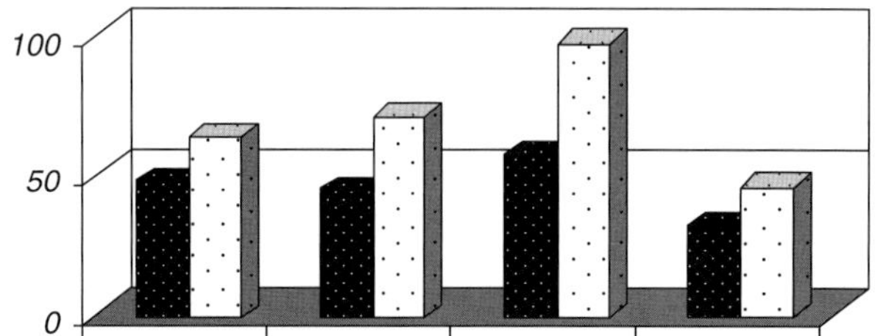

	MTT	TTP	CBF	CBV
■ Pre OP	48	43,9	47,89	32,46
□ Post OP	63,09	70,65	96,87	45

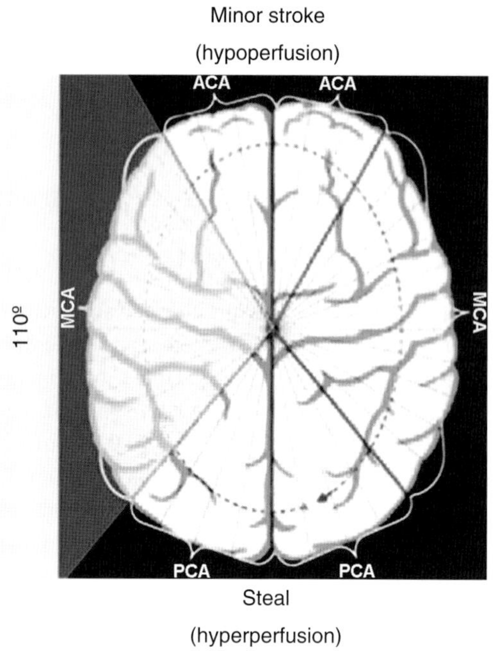

Fig. 3 Results of the segregated 110° expanded MCA territory pre- and postoperatively in patients 1 and 10 with conspicuous differences in comparison to the holo-hemispheric results

Discussion

Lowering blood pressure to normal or upper-normal values in the early postoperative period after intracranial surgery is generally accepted practice. In patients with chronic atherosclerotic cerebral occlusive disease, this lowering can cause hypoperfusion. However, in these patients cerebrovascular reconstructive surgery can cause a rapid increase in CBF resulting in cerebral hyperperfusion. Hyperperfusion syndrome incidentally occurs in patients after carotid endarterectomy [12] or removal of an arteriovenous malformation. Also patients with STA-MCA anastomosis, which provides in general low-flow revascularization, can sustain symptomatic hyperperfusion syndrome with unilateral headaches, facial and ocular pain, focal symptoms secondary to cerebral edema [3–5, 8], seizures or intracranial hemorrhage [12]. CBF is described to increase greatly in the first 24 h after revascularization procedures with a second maximum on day 5. Between these days, cerebral edema reduces the total blood flow volume [7].

During the first hours after revascularization procedures patients are at high risk of developing an unnoticed hypo- or hyperperfusion due to the lack of alertness after general anesthesia. Inhalation anesthesia itself raises the CBF, and after removal of the endotracheal tubes, cerebral blood flow also increases [1]. During this time perfusion parameters and information about the postoperative intracranial status are required in order to adapt blood pressure levels. Online techniques such as regional cerebral blood flow [15], laser Doppler flowmeter [7] or brain-tissue oxygenation measurements [10] have the advantage of providing permanent information, but the monitored brain region is small, the procedure is invasive, and additional information is missing. Well-established examinations like perfusion MRI, SPECT or PET [16] involve a transfer, sometimes into another building, and perfusion studies are time consuming. In contrast, PCT is a fast technique, and a CT scanner is frequently available close to the ICU. Results are available immediately, and additional information is provided (i.e., about hemorrhage, infarction, edema).

The goal of this study was to identify unexpected cerebral perfusion changes using PCT in the early postoperative period in comparison to preoperative PCT in order to use these results for planning further diagnostic or therapeutic procedures. Holo-hemispheric changes could be detected in all patients. In 80% of the patients an expected increase of CBF and CBV and shortened TTP and MTT were diagnosed. In two patients holo-hemispheric PCT identified 50% respectively 100% unexpected changes in the four perfusion parameters. These patients with clinical aggravation were further examined. A detailed analysis of the MCA territory was performed. Patient 1 presented with an increase of holo-hemispheric CBF and CBV, but also with a delayed TTP and MTT. In the MCA territory, TTP and MTT were also prolonged; however, CBF and CBV decreased. These changes could be identified as hypoperfusion of the MCA territory. A subsequent CT scan revealed a minor stroke in a corresponding vascular territory. Patient 10 presented with an unexpected decrease of holo-hemispheric CBF and CBV as well as prolonged TTP and MTT. Closer inspection of the MCA territory confirmed the delay of TTP and MTT. A significant increase of CBF and CBV was detected. With holo-hemispheric reduced perfusion and considerably increased CBF and CBV in the MCA territory, this was interpreted as hyperperfusion with the steal phenomenon. The following imaging detected small borderzone infarctions, which supported the assumption of hyperperfusion with the steal effect. Thus, unexpected changes of two or more holo-hemispheric perfusion parameters with a close examination of the subdivided MCA territories can be suggestive of hypo- or hyperperfusion after bypass surgery.

Conclusion

This pilot study demonstrates that early PCT parameters can provide immediate and detailed information about the hemodynamic situation after cerebral bypass surgery. Furthermore, PCT analysis seems to have a predictive value in this patient population regarding the morbidity due to hypo- or hyperperfusion. However, this still needs to be supported by prospective investigations with a larger patient cohort.

Conflict of interest statement We declare that we have no conflict of interest.

References

1. Bruder N, Pellissier D, Grillot P, Gouin F (2002) Cerebral hyperemia during recovery from general anesthesia in neurosurgical patients. Anesth Analg 94:650–654
2. Derdeyn CP, Videen TO, Simmons NR, Yundt KD, Fritsch SM, Grubb RL Jr, Powers WJ (1999) Count-based PET method for predicting ischemic stroke in patients with symptomatic carotid arterial occlusion. Radiology 212:499–506
3. Fujimura M, Kaneta T, Mugikura S, Shimizu H, Tominaga T (2007) Temporary neurologic deterioration due to cerebral hyperperfusion after superficial temporal artery-middle cerebral artery anastomosis in patients with adult-onset Moyamoya disease. Surg Neurol 67:273–282
4. Fujimura M, Mugikura S, Kaneta T, Shimizu H, Tominaga T (2008) Efficacy of superficial temporal artery-middle cerebral artery anastomosis with routine postoperative cerebral blood flow measurement during the acute stage in childhood Moyamoya disease. Childs Nerv Syst 24:827–832
5. Fukuda T, Ogasawara K, Kobayashi M, Komoribayashi N, Endo H, Inoue T, Kuzu Y, Nishimoto H, Terasaki K, Ogawa A (2007) Prediction of cerebral hyperperfusion after carotid endarterectomy using cerebral blood volume measurement by perfusion-weighted MR imaging compared with single-photon emission CT. AJNR Am J Neuroradiol 28:737–742
6. Furukawa M, Kashiwagi S, Matsunaga N, Suzuki M, Kishimoto K, Shirao S (2002) Evaluation of cerebral perfusion parameters measured by perfusion CT in chronic cerebral ischemia: comparison with xenon CT. J Comput Assist Tomogr 26:272–278
7. Gesang DZ, Zhang D, Zhao JZ, Wang S, YI Z, Wang R, Sun JJ, Meng Z (2009) Laser Doppler flowmeter study on regional cerebral blood flow in early stage after standard superficial temporal artery-middle cerebral artery bypass surgery for Moyamoya disease. Chin Med J 122:2412–2418
8. Heros RC, Scott RM, Kister JP, Ackerman RH, Conner ES (1984) Temporary neurological deterioration after extracranial-intracranial bypass. Neurosurgery 15:178–185
9. Hoffmann WE, Charbel FT, Abood C, Ausman JI (1997) Regional ischemia during bypass surgery. Surg Neurol 47:455–459
10. Matsuda H, Higashi S, Kinuya K, Tsuji S, Nozaki J, Sumiya H, Hisada K, Yamashita J (1991) SPECT evaluation of brain perfusion reserve by acetazolamide test using Tc-99 m HMPAO. Clin Nucl Med 16:572–579
11. Nakamizo A, Inoue T, Kikawa Y, Uda K, Hirata Y, Okamura K, Yasaka M, Okada Y (2009) Postoperative evaluation of changes in extracranial-intracranial bypass graft using superficial temporal artery duplex ultrasonography. AJNR Am J Neuroradiol 30:900–905
12. Piepgras DG, Morgan MK, Sundt TM Jr, Yanagihara T, Mussman LM (1988) Intracerebral hemorrhage after carotid endarterectomy. J Neurosurg 68:532–536
13. Schmiedek P, Piepgras A, Leinsinger G, Kirsch CM, Einhäupl K (1994) Improvement of cerebrovascular reserve capacity by EC-IC arterial bypass surgery in patients with ICA occlusion and haemodynamic cerebral ischemia. J Neurosurg 81:236–244
14. Turowski B, Hanggi D, Wittsack HJ, Beck A, Aurich V (2006) Computerized analysis of brain perfusion parameter images. Rofo 179:525–529
15. Vajkocy P, Roth H, Horn P, Lucke T, Thomé C, Hubner U, Martin GT, Zappletal C, Klar E, Schilling L, Schmiedek P (2000) Continuous monitoring of regional cerebral blood flow: experimental and clinical validation of a novel thermal diffusion microprobe. J Neurosurg 93:265–274
16. Wanebo JE, Amin-Hanjani S, Boyd C, Peery T (2005) Assessing success after cerebral revascularization for ischemia. Skull Base 15:215–227
17. Wittsack HJ, Kleiser R, Cohnen M, Moedder U (2004) CT-perfusion imaging with deconvolution analysis by singular value decomposition: misuse your old CT-scanner for cerebral perfusion analysis. Congress of the Radiological Society of North America RSNA, Chicago. http://rsna2004.rsna.org/rsna2004/V2004/conference/event_display.cfm?em_id=4410557. Accessed 2004
18. Woitzik J, Horn P, Vajkocy P, Schmiedek P (2005) Intraoperative control of extracranial-intracranial bypass patency by near-infrared indocyanine green videoangiography. J Neurosurg 102:692–698
19. Yonas H, Smith HA, Durham SR, Pentheny SL, Johnson DW (1993) Increased stroke risk predicted by compromised cerebral blood flow reactivity. J Neurosurg 79:483–489

Genetic and Clinical Characteristics of Moyamoya Disease in Europeans

Boris Krischek, Hidetoshi Kasuya, Nadia Khan, Marcos Tatagiba, Constantin Roder, and Markus Kraemer

Abstract The European form of Moyamoya disease clearly differs from the Asian form. Clinically the timing of vasculopathy onset and a lower rate of hemorrhage are striking as compared to the Asian Moyamoya disease.

Single nucleotide polymorphisms that play a role in atherosclerosis, vascular growth and transformation processes have been found to be associated with the European form. Candidate gene associations found in Asian patients could not be replicated in European patients.

To elucidate the characteristics, we describe the clinical features as well as the genetic findings that we have found in our combined cohorts of European patients.

Keywords European · Genetics · Hemorrhage · Ischemia · Moyamoya disease

B. Krischek (✉), M. Tatagiba, and C. Roder
Department of Neurosurgery, University of Tübingen, Hoppe-Seyler-Strasse 3, 72076 Tübingen, Germany
e-mail: krischek@gmail.com

H. Kasuya
Division of Neurosurgery, Medical Center East, Tokyo Women's Medical University, 2-1-10 Nishiogu, Arakawa-ku, Tokyo 116-8567, Japan

N. Khan
Moyamoya Clinic, Children's University Hospital Zurich, Steinwiesstrasse 75, 8032 Zurich, Switzerland

M. Kraemer
Department of Neurology, Alfried Krupp von Bohlen und Halbach Hospital, Essen, Germany

Introduction

Up to now, there is only limited knowledge about Moyamoya disease, especially in Europeans. Differences or similarities in disease presentation in Asians and Caucasians are a source of scientific debate, and mechanisms of pathophysiology are still widely unknown. In several articles from Europe, there is also disagreement about whether analysis of Caucasian patients should include all patients with Moyamoya angiopathy (e.g., Moyamoya disease, Moyamoya syndrome and unilateral Moyamoya angiopathy) or should be restricted to patients with idiopathic Moyamoya disease only [17, 18, 30].

Until recently there have been no genetic studies on Moyamoya disease in Europe. In an attempt to understand the molecular pathomechanism of the disease, we performed several candidate gene association studies to replicate previous findings performed in Asian patients, and also tried to find parallels to other diseases such as atherosclerosis and to known histopathological changes in Moyamoya disease.

Epidemiology

Moyamoya disease shows a remarkable difference in region and ethnicity [28]. It is mostly found in Asians, especially in Japan and Korea. The incidence in Japan has been reported to be 0.35/100,000, whereas a questionnaire-based inquiry revealed a frequency of one-tenth of that (0.03) in Europe [1, 28, 30, 31].

Asian epidemiological surveys have shown a female predominance ranging from 1.8:1 in sporadic to 5:1 in familial cases of MMD [20]. In North American studies with cases of various ethnic backgrounds, female predominance of around 2:1 was reported [3, 10, 11]. In a recent German study with 21 Caucasian patients with idiopathic Moyamoya disease, a female predominance of 4.25:1 was noted [18], whereas in our studies with 40 patients from central Europe it was 2.1:1 [24, 25].

T. Tsukahara et al. (eds.), *Trends in Neurovascular Surgery*, Acta Neurochirurgica Supplementum, Vol. 112,
DOI: 10.1007/978-3-7091-0661-7_6, © Springer-Verlag/Wien 2011

Clinical Characteristics

Due to rarity of the disease in Europe, the different inclusion criteria of patients in studies and the lack of any systematic prospective multi-center survey, there is some confusion and debate about the disease presentation and age distribution in Europeans.

Even if including North American studies in the characterization of the disease in Caucasians, this is difficult because of multi-ethnic and heterogeneous cohorts of patients with Moyamoya disease and Moyamoya syndrome. In 1998, Chiu et al. reported 22 Caucasian Americans with Moyamoya disease and described several differences between disease presentation in the United States and in Japan [3]. Another Caucasian cohort with 23 Americans was reviewed by Hallemeier et al. in 2006 [11]. Recently, a group at Stanford published an analysis on 329 American patients of whom 59% were of Caucasian origin [10].

Most authors in Europe and North America describe a considerable difference in clinical disease presentation between Caucasian and the Asian Moyamoya patients [30]. In a German cohort of 21 adult patients with idiopathic Moyamoya disease, all had presented with ischemic symptom onset [18], whereas most adults with Asian background present with hemorrhage [26, 30]. In the German study, only 1 of the 21 patients had experienced subarachnoid hemorrhage [18]. In Chiu's North American study, only 13% of the adult patients had suffered intracranial hemorrhages (17% overall) [3]. Another US multicenter study by Numaguchi et al. revealed a similarly low prevalence of intracranial hemorrhage (14%) [22]. In Hawaii, the proportion of Moyamoya patients presenting with intracranial hemorrhage is higher (29%), but the majority of patients included in that study were of Asian ethnicity [7]. Also in Hallemeier's study most Caucasian patients presented with ischemic symptoms [11]. However, recently Guzman et al. compared the presenting symptoms of their 69 American patients of Asian ethnic background with 137 Caucasian American Moyamoya patients and found no statistically significant difference in the incidence of ischemic events such as stroke (67% versus 65%) or transient ischemic attacks (61% versus 67%) [9, 10]. The rate of hemorrhagic presentation was 24% in Asian Americans compared to 16% in Caucasian Americans, but this did not reach statistical significance ($p=0.08$) [9, 10]. However, in contrast to former data [26], in a novel Japanese study with 267 patients, intracranial hemorrhage was present in 21.3% and ischemic stroke in 56.9% [1]. Asian pediatric patients present with ischemic symptoms, and hemorrhages are very rare [26]. It is likely that ischemic events appear soon after the onset of the arterial occlusion or narrowing [18]. In Asia, this most frequently occurs in childhood, and the frequency of transient ischemic attacks and cerebral infarctions is highest at that time [18, 27]. In accordance with another American study [11], a higher risk of recurrent ischemic events within the first 2 years after symptom onset was observed in the German cohort [18]. This may reflect an improvement in collateral flow over time. The increased risk of hemorrhages in Asian adults may be the consequence of an extensive network of fragile Moyamoya collaterals that have developed over decades since their childhood [18].

In Asian patients the age distribution shows a peak in childhood at 5 years of age with ischemic symptoms, and another peak of disease presentation in adulthood between the ages of 45 and 49 [1]. Hallemeier et al. concluded that differences in presentation between North American and Asian patients may be related to the timing of onset of the occlusive vasculopathy and supposed that in Caucasians disease onset may be more frequent in young adults [11]. However, the age distribution in Caucasian patients is uncertain. While the pediatric age peak was lacking in two American Studies and a European study [3, 11, 18], other groups in Europe and the US found no difference in age distributions between Caucasian and Asian patients [9, 10, 30].

Additional symptoms in European or Caucasian Moyamoya disease are mostly neglected in the literature. However, limited data suggest that additional symptoms such as headache and epilepsy are also frequent in European patients [18]. Judging by our own clinical experience, it is important to ask adult European patients if there were triggering factors for their ischemic symptoms [18]. In Asian patients ischemic events are associated with hyperventilation [21].

Little is known about the natural course of Moyamoya disease in Europeans, whose 5-year Kaplan-Meier risk of recurrent stroke was reported to be 80.95% after the first ischemic event for all patients [18]. In an American study patients with bilateral involvement presenting with ischemic symptoms were at the highest risk of subsequent stroke (an 82% 5-year risk of developing a stroke with medical treatment after the first symptom occurred) [11]. It was discussed whether there is a phase after which the disease can be considered quiescent or "burned out" [3, 18]. However, both Asian and North American series describe an inevitable disease progression [13, 14, 19]. Even though operative and conservative treatment has never been systematically evaluated in European patients [18], it is largely agreed upon that in most cases a revascularization procedure is advisable and the most beneficial therapeutic concept [4, 5, 9, 12, 15, 16, 29].

Recently, an American study described similar features in idiopathic occlusive disease of the basal arteries without Moyamoya collaterals compared to Moyamoya disease [2, 6]. This leads to the question whether unilateral Moyamoya angiopathy, idiopathic Moyamoya disease and occlusive disease of the basal arteries represent individual entities. Nevertheless, for European patients who have the Moyamoya phenomenon, it is crucial to perform detailed differential diagnostic procedures to differentiate among idiopathic Moyamoya disease, Moyamoya syndrome and other occlusive diseases, as each entity may require a different form of therapy [17].

Genetic Findings in Europeans

Several genetic studies of Asian Moyamoya disease patients have been published in the last years. To date no single gene has been associated with the disease, possibly indicating that it is a multigenic occurrence. In a recent review of all data that had been published so far, it was evident that candidate gene associations found in Asian individuals could not be replicated [23].

We conducted a series of single nucleotide polymorphism analyses in which we examined 40 MMD patients of central European background and 68 healthy controls. The mean age of onset of MMD-related symptoms was 15.4 years of age.

Atherosclerosis

In our first study we genotyped 17 single nucleotide polymorphisms in or adjacent to 11 genes (*ELN, LIMK1, CDKN2A/B, CXCL12, Pseudogene ENSG00000197218, PSRC1, MTHFD1L, SMAD3, MIA3, PDGF-B, TIMP2*) [24].

We found an association of one SNP (rs599839 [A/G], OR = 2.17, 95% CI = 1.17, 4.05; $p = 0.01$) with the risk allele G located in the 3′ UTR region of the *PSRC-1* gene. Three further SNPs (rs8326, rs34208922, rs501120) in or adjacent to the genes *ELN* and *CXCL12* showed tendencies to risk alleles with p-values between 0.1 and 0.2, but did not reach statistical significance in our cohort. The risk allele G ($p = 0.014$) of the rs599839SNP [A/G] SNP is located on chromosome 1p13.3 in the 3′ UTR region of the *PSRC-1* gene (proline/serine-rich coiled-coil 1) and is close to the *CELSR2* (cadherin, EGF LAG seven-pass G-type receptor 2) gene. This genetic locus is at the telomeric portion of a 150-kbp segment that has been described to be associated with LDL cholesterol levels in genome-wide association studies (GWAS). LDL cholesterol is known to play an important role among the risk factors for the genesis of atherosclerotic lesions. These results indicate a possible parallel of common processes in the genesis of Moyamoya and atherosclerotic disease [24].

TGFB1 and PDGFRB

We analyzed the DNA of patients with Moyamoya disease for single nucleotide polymorphisms in and upstream of the genes for previously described associated cytokines and growth factors [25]. Thirteen SNPs were genotyped in or upstream to four genes (*bFGF*, *CRABP1*, *PDGFRB*, *TGFB1*). We found an association of two SNPs: rs382861 [A/C] ($p = 0.0373$, OR = 1.81, 95% CI = 1.03–3.17) in the promoter region of *PDGFRB* and rs1800471[C/G] ($p = 0.0345$, OR = 7.65, 95% CI = 0.97–59.95) located in the first exon of *TGFB1*.

TGFB1 and *PDGFRB* are involved in vascular growth and transformation processes, which may play a role in the development of Moyamoya disease.

ACTA2

Recently, the coincidence of mutations in *ACTA2* (vascular smooth muscle cell-specific isoform of α-actin) in families with thoracic aortic aneurysms and dissections (TAAD) and Moyamoya disease was reported in patients of Northern European descent and a positive family history of TAAD and MMD [8]. In this study, we analyzed the nine exons of the *ACTA2* gene in central European patients with non-familial MMD, aiming to replicate previously described genetic findings and possibly identify further mutations. DNA sequencing of the nine exons and flanking intronic regions of *ACTA2* was performed in 39 MMD patients with no family history of MMD or TAAD and 68 healthy controls of central European descent. One new mutation in exon 6 of *ACTA2* was found in one patient with MMD. We were not able to detect the previously described mutations (unpublished data).

Conclusions

There are several clinical differences between European and Asian patients diagnosed with Moyamoya disease. This in itself may already be a sign of the different genetic components that play a role in the disease's formation in people of different ethnicities.

Further analyses in larger European cohorts and replication in patients of different ethnicities may lead to possible early detection of patients at risk of developing Moyamoya disease and subsequently to an understanding of the disease's pathophysiology.

Conflict of interest statement We declare that we have no conflict of interest.

References

1. Baba T, Houkin K, Kuroda S (2008) Novel epidemiological features of Moyamoya disease. J Neurol Neurosurg Psychiatry 79:900–904
2. Braun KP, Bulder MM, Chabrier S, Kirkham FJ, Uiterwaal CS, Tardieu M, Sebire G (2009) The course and outcome of unilateral intracranial arteriopathy in 79 children with ischaemic stroke. Brain 132:544–557
3. Chiu D, Shedden P, Grotta JC (1998) Clinical features of Moyamoya disease in the United States. Stroke 29:1347–1351
4. Czabanka M, Pena-Tapia P, Schubert GA, Woitzik J, Horn P, Schmiedek P, Vajkoczy P (2009) Clinical implications of cortical

microvasculature in adult Moyamoya disease. J Cereb Blood Flow Metab 29:1383–1387
5. Czabanka M, Vajkoczy P, Schmiedek P, Horn P (2009) Age-dependent revascularization patterns in the treatment of Moyamoya disease in a European patient population. Neurosurg Focus 26:E9
6. Goyal MS, Hallemeier CL, Zipfel GJ, Rich KM, Grubb RL Jr, Chicoine MR, Moran CJ, Cross DT 3rd, Dacey RG Jr, Derdeyn CP (2010) Clinical features and outcome in North American adults with idiopathic basal arterial occlusive disease without moyamoya collaterals. Neurosurgery 67:278–285
7. Graham JF, Matoba A (1997) A survey of Moyamoya disease in Hawaii. Clin Neurol Neurosurg 99(Suppl 2):S31–S35
8. Guo DC, Papke CL, Tran-Fadulu V, Regalado ES, Avidan N, Johnson RJ, Kim DH, Pannu H, Willing MC, Sparks E, Pyeritz RE, Singh MN, Dalman RL, Grotta JC, Marian AJ, Boerwinkle EA, Frazier LQ, LeMaire SA, Coselli JS, Estrera AL, Safi HJ, Veeraraghavan S, Muzny DM, Wheeler DA, Willerson JT, Yu RK, Shete SS, Scherer SE, Raman CS, Buja LM, Milewicz DM (2009) Mutations in smooth muscle alpha-actin (ACTA2) cause coronary artery disease, stroke, and Moyamoya disease, along with thoracic aortic disease. Am J Hum Genet 84:617–627
9. Guzman R, Khan N, Steinberg G (2010) Moyamoya disease in North America. In: Cho B-K, Tominaga T (eds) Moyamoya disease update. Springer, New York
10. Guzman R, Lee M, Achrol A, Bell-Stephens T, Kelly M, Do HM, Marks MP, Steinberg GK (2009) Clinical outcome after 450 revascularization procedures for Moyamoya disease. Clinical article. J Neurosurg 111:927–935
11. Hallemeier CL, Rich KM, Grubb RL Jr, Chicoine MR, Moran CJ, Cross DT 3rd, Zipfel GJ, Dacey RG Jr, Derdeyn CP (2006) Clinical features and outcome in North American adults with moyamoya phenomenon. Stroke 37:1490–1496
12. Hanggi D, Mehrkens JH, Schmid-Elsaesser R, Steiger HJ (2008) Results of direct and indirect revascularisation for adult European patients with Moyamoya angiopathy. Acta Neurochir Suppl 103:119–122
13. Imaizumi T, Hayashi K, Saito K, Osawa M, Fukuyama Y (1998) Long-term outcomes of pediatric Moyamoya disease monitored to adulthood. Pediatr Neurol 18:321–325
14. Kelly ME, Bell-Stephens TE, Marks MP, Do HM, Steinberg GK (2006) Progression of unilateral Moyamoya disease: a clinical series. Cerebrovasc Dis 22:109–115
15. Khan N, Schuknecht B, Boltshauser E, Capone A, Buck A, Imhof HG, Yonekawa Y (2003) Moyamoya disease and Moyamoya syndrome: experience in Europe; choice of revascularisation procedures. Acta Neurochir (Wien) 145:1061–1071; discussion 1071
16. Khan N, Yonekawa Y (2008) Moyamoya angiopathy in Europe: the beginnings in Zurich, practical lessons learned, increasing awareness and future perspectives. Acta Neurochir Suppl 103: 127–130
17. Kraemer M, Berlit P (2010) Primary central nervous system vasculitis and Moyamoya disease: similarities and differences. J Neurol 257:816–819
18. Kraemer M, Heienbrok W, Berlit P (2008) Moyamoya disease in Europeans. Stroke 39:3193–3200
19. Kuroda S, Ishikawa T, Houkin K, Nanba R, Hokari M, Iwasaki Y (2005) Incidence and clinical features of disease progression in adult Moyamoya disease. Stroke 36:2148–2153
20. Kuroda S, Iwasaki Y (2006) Current review of familial Moyamoya disease. Nippon Rinsho 64(Suppl 8):750–754
21. Kuwabara Y, Ichiya Y, Sasaki M, Yoshida T, Masuda K, Matsushima T, Fukui M (1997) Response to hypercapnia in moyamoya disease. Cerebrovascular response to hypercapnia in pediatric and adult patients with Moyamoya disease. Stroke 28:701–707
22. Numaguchi Y, Gonzalez CF, Davis PC, Monajati A, Afshani E, Chang J, Sutton CL, Lee RR, Shibata DK (1997) Moyamoya disease in the United States. Clin Neurol Neurosurg 99(Suppl 2): S26–S30
23. Roder C, Nayak NR, Khan N, Tatagiba M, Inoue I, Krischek B (2010) Genetics of Moyamoya disease. J Hum Genet 55(11): 711–716
24. Roder C, Peters V, Kasuya H, Nishizawa T, Takehara Y, Berg D, Schulte C, Khan N, Tatagiba M, Krischek B (2010) Common genetic polymorphisms in Moyamoya and atherosclerotic disease in Europeans. Childs Nerv Syst 27(2):245–252
25. Roder C, Peters V, Kasuya H, Nishizawa T, Takehara Y, Berg D, Schulte C, Khan N, Tatagiba M, Krischek B (2010) Polymorphisms in TGFB1 and PDGFRB are associated with Moyamoya disease in European patients. Acta Neurochir (Wien) 152(12):2153–2160
26. Suzuki J, Kodama N (1983) Moyamoya disease: a review. Stroke 14:104–109
27. Tagawa T, Naritomi H, Mimaki T, Yabuuchi H, Sawada T (1987) Regional cerebral blood flow, clinical manifestations, and age in children with Moyamoya disease. Stroke 18:906–910
28. Uchino K, Johnston SC, Becker KJ, Tirschwell DL (2005) Moyamoya disease in Washington state and California. Neurology 65:956–958
29. Vajkoczy P (2009) Moyamoya disease: collateralization is everything. Cerebrovasc Dis 28:258
30. Yonekawa Y, Fandino J, Hug M, Wiesli M, Fujioka M, Khan N (2010) Moyamoya angiopathy in Europe. In: Cho B-K, Tominaga T (eds) Moyamoya disease update. Springer, New York
31. Yonekawa Y, Ogata N, Kaku Y, Taub E, Imhof HG (1997) Moyamoya disease in Europe, past and present status. Clin Neurol Neurosurg 99(Suppl 2):S58–S60

Effect of Mouth Opening on Bypass Function After Combined Revascularization for Moyamoya Disease

C.F. Freyschlag[‡], M. Seiz[‡], M. A. Brockmann, J. Scharf, R.W. Stier, G.A. Schubert, C. Thomé, and P. Schmiedek

Abstract Moyamoya disease represents a rare steno-occlusive disease of the internal carotid artery (ICA) with a reactive and pathological basal network of collateral vessels. It may lead to ischemic stroke or intracerebral hemorrhage. Treatment options are either direct or indirect revascularization procedures or a combination thereof. Specialized centers report sufficient revascularization in most patients and low complication rates.

Between 2005 and 2008, direct extra-intracranial bypass surgery in combination with encephalomyosynangiosis (EMS) was performed in 71 Moyamoya patients at the Mannheim University Medical Center.

Following one case of reversible neurological deficits associated with mouth opening, we prospectively evaluated the effect of mouth opening on bypass function in this patient and four further consecutive patients by digital subtraction angiography.

Three out of five patients showed alterations in bypass patency upon mouth opening. The obstruction was located at the junction of the bypass and the temporal muscle. Two temporary occlusions and one case of decreased flow were observed. One patient demonstrated reversible hemiparesis and aphasia.

C.F. Freyschlag (✉), M. Seiz, G.A. Schubert, and C. Thomé
Department of Neurosurgery, University Medical Center Mannheim, University of Heidelberg, Heidelberg, Germany and
Department of Neurosurgery, University Hospital Innsbruck, Innsbruck Medical University, Innsbruck, Austria
e-mail: christian.freyschlag@i-med.ac.at

R.W. Stier and P. Schmiedek
Department of Neurosurgery, University Medical Center Mannheim, University of Heidelberg, Heidelberg, Germany

M.A. Brockmann and J. Scharf
Department of Neuroradiology, University Medical Center Mannheim, University of Heidelberg, Heidelberg, Germany

Keywords Direct indirect revascularization · Encephalomyosynangiosis · Extra-intracranial bypass · Mouth opening · Moyamoya disease

Introduction

Moyamoya disease is a rare idiopathic vascular disease with progressive stenosis or occlusion of the internal carotid artery and dependent vessels. First described in 1957 by Takeuchi [24] as a bilateral hypoplasia of the internal carotid arteries, the pathognomonic dilated collateral network was first described by Suzuki [23], who named the disease after the Japanese term "moyamoya" for puff of smoke. Despite the unknown etiology, the significantly higher incidence in the Asian population [25] strongly suggests a genetic coherence. Moyamoya conditions are found with an estimated incidence of 0.08 per 100,000 in Western populations [3, 26].

Treatment options are either medical therapy or surgery. Conservative strategies have been used in patients with a high perioperative risk profile or relatively mild course of disease. Medical treatment consists of antiplatelet agents or symptomatic treatment (eg., treatment of headaches).

Surgical treatment of patients with Moyamoya typically uses revascularization procedures such as indirect or direct anastomoses [2, 5, 9–11, 14, 15, 17, 21, 22]. Bilateral direct revascularization with a combined procedure of extra-intracranial bypass and modified encephalomyosynangiosis for the hemisphere with the smaller cerebrovascular reserve capacity and EMS for the contralateral hemisphere is standard treatment in our center. The technique is modified by direct guidance of the donor vessel through the fibers of the EMS instead of diverting it around the muscle.

[‡]Authors Freyschlag CF and Seiz M contributed equally to this study.

Materials and Methods

Following one incidence of temporary neurological deficit in a combined revascularized patient, we did extensive diagnostics and prospectively analyzed four further adult patients treated for Moyamoya disease within routinely scheduled follow-up.

All subjects underwent six-vessel digital subtraction angiography plus selective external carotid injection with opened and closed mouth. Furthermore the patients were clinically examined with provocation by mouth opening. Angiographic studies of these patients were analyzed by an experienced interventional neuroradiologist (J.S.).

Neurological examination consisted of pronator drift test and Janda's muscle examination [13]. None of the patients showed neurological deficits upon the beginning of examination. Provocation by active mouth opening for 2 min revealed a right side hemiparesis of brachial predominance and aphasia in one patient. Both symptoms fully recovered after several minutes.

Three out of five patients showed alterations in bypass patency due to mouth opening. We found two complete occlusions of the direct anastomosis (Fig. 1). One patient showed a decrease of flow in the donor vessel. Two patients showed no affection of the bypass.

Results

Five patients (3 females, 2 males) with a mean age of 56 years (47–63 years) underwent routinely scheduled digital subtraction angiography and clinical examination. The mean age at treatment was 52.8 years (43–58 years); surgery was performed with uneventful postoperative course between 2005 and 2008 at the Mannheim University Medical Center. Treatment consisted of combined revascularization of the dominant hemisphere and contralateral stand-alone EMS. We found ten revascularized hemispheres [5 combined (3 left, 2 right) and 5 contralateral EMS].

Discussion

The etiology of Moyamoya disease is still unknown, but the vasculopathy seems to be unresponsive to drug therapy [4]. The use of microsurgery and the implementation of extra-intracranial bypass surgery by Yasargil and Donaghy [6] in 1967 led us to an effective treatment of Moyamoya disease.

According to Choi et al. [4], patients with Moyamoya disease benefit greatly from cerebral revascularization compared to the natural history. The term indirect revascularization includes several different techniques of cerebral

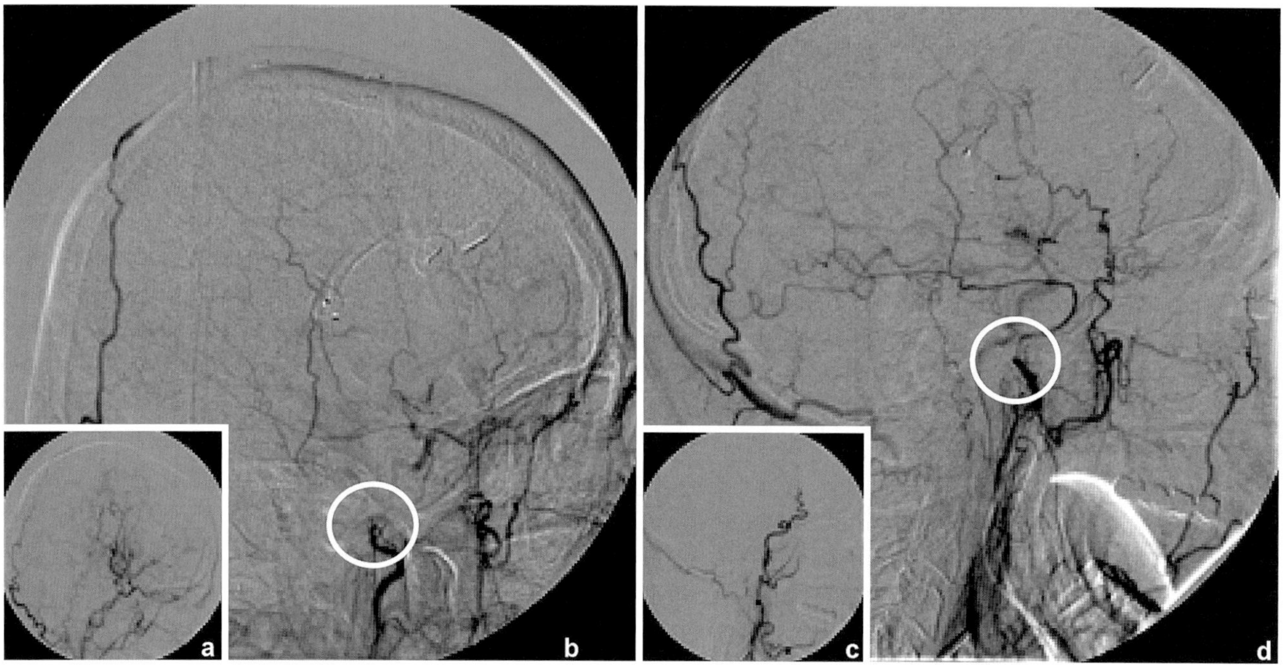

Fig. 1 (**a**) Digital subtraction angiography of a 56-year-old patient with complete occlusion of the bypass while opening the mouth, during which the patient suffered brachial predominant hemiparesis and aphasia. (**b**) Same patient without mouth opening, showing a patent bypass. (**c**) DSA of a 63-year-old patient with another complete occlusion of the bypass vessel, without any neurological impairment. (**d**) Same patient without mouth opening, again showing a patent bypass

synangiosis with the dura, temporal muscle, arteries or combinations of them [2, 8, 11, 12, 15–17]. Indirect procedures are disadvantageous for providing immediate perfusion to the oxygen-deprived areas, whereas direct extra-intracranial bypass can fail in the long-term course. Combined revascularization leads to immediate re-perfusion and long-lasting restoration of the cerebral oxygen supply.

Age-dependent revascularization patterns are discussed by Czabanka et al. [5], showing that combined revascularization with direct anastomosis and bilateral encephalomyosynangiosis is safe and efficient. Whereas in an adult population direct anastomosis showed marginally better angiographic results compared to indirect encephalomyosynangiosis, contrary results are seen in a pediatric cohort. Matsushima et al. showed that combined revascularization is superior to indirect procedures alone [17]. The major difference compared to published data is that our technique guides the donor vessel directly through the EMS instead of diverting the bypass around the muscle fibers, which notably shortens the bypass vessel length. It further simplifies applying the end-to-side anastomosis. Overall complication rates with this modified technique are as low as those published for combined revascularization [2, 5, 8, 20].

Overall postoperative complication rates are low and depend on the chosen procedure [11]. Encephalomyosyngiosis requires a wider craniotomy than direct anastomosis only and may lead to a mass effect because of muscle swelling or hematoma [7, 19, 21, 27]. The complication rates of direct anastomosis for Moyamoya disease [18] are equal to those for standard extra-intracranial bypass [1, 11].

Up to now, secondary occlusion of direct revascularization due to mouth opening has not been reported after operative treatment of Moyamoya disease or extra-intracranial bypass surgery in general.

Two of five patients in our cohort showed complete obstruction of the bypass while opening the mouth. In combined revascularization, the donor vessel is guided through the fibers of the temporal muscle. Therefore, we propose that axial extension of the fiber orientation leads to compression and furthermore occlusion of the graft. One patient showed neurological deficits because of the combination of occluded bypass and poor EMS function, whereas in the other patient the EMS was sufficiently vascularized.

We conclude that in the absence of prospective comparative evaluation of revascularization patterns in Moyamoya disease, the combination of STA-MCA bypass and encephalomyosynangiosis leads to effective treatment [2]. We also think that longitudinal splitting of the muscle graft with the encephalomyosynangiosis technique can be helpful in providing sufficient indirect revascularization and is advantageous because of its relation to the donor vessel. This modification of surgical technique is the subject of our ongoing research.

Conflict of interest statement We declare that we have no conflict of interest.

References

1. Andrews BT, Chater NL, Weinstein PR (1985) Extracranial-intracranial arterial bypass for middle cerebral artery stenosis and occlusion. Operative results in 65 cases. J Neurosurg 6:831–838. doi:10.3171/jns.1985.62.6.0831
2. Baaj AA, Agazzi S, Sayed ZA, Toledo M, Spetzler RF, van Loveren H (2009) Surgical management of Moyamoya disease: a review. Neurosurg Focus 4:E7. doi:10.3171/2009.01.FOCUS08293
3. Burke GM, Burke AM, Sherma AK, Hurley MC, Batjer HH, Bendok BR (2009) Moyamoya disease: a summary. Neurosurg Focus 4:E11. doi:10.3171/2009.1.FOCUS08310
4. Choi JU, Kim DS, Kim EY, Lee KC (1997) Natural history of Moyamoya disease: comparison of activity of daily living in surgery and nonsurgery groups. Clin Neurol Neurosurg 99(Suppl 2): S11–S18
5. Czabanka M, Vajkoczy P, Schmiedek P, Horn P (2009) Age-dependent revascularization patterns in the treatment of Moyamoya disease in a European patient population. Neurosurg Focus 4:E9. doi:10.3171/2009.1.FOCUS08298
6. Donaghy RM (1972) Neurologic surgery. Surg Gynecol Obstet 2:269–270
7. Fujimura M, Kaneta T, Shimizu H, Tominaga T (2009) Cerebral ischemia owing to compression of the brain by swollen temporal muscle used for encephalo-myo-synangiosis in Moyamoya disease. Neurosurg Rev 2:245–249. doi:10.1007/s10143-009-0184-6; discussion 249
8. Fung LW, Thompson D, Ganesan V (2005) Revascularisation surgery for paediatric Moyamoya: a review of the literature. Childs Nerv Syst 5:358–364. doi:10.1007/s00381-004-1118-9
9. Golby AJ, Marks MP, Thompson RC, Steinberg GK (1999) Direct and combined revascularization in pediatric Moyamoya disease. Neurosurgery 1:50–58; discussion 58–60
10. Gratzl O, Schmiedek P, Spetzler R, Steinhoff H, Marguth F (1976) Clinical experience with extra-intracranial arterial anastomosis in 65 cases. J Neurosurg 3:313–324. doi:10.3171/jns.1976.44.3.0313
11. Guzman R, Lee M, Achrol A, Bell-Stephens T, Kelly M, Do HM et al (2009) Clinical outcome after 450 revascularization procedures for Moyamoya disease. Clinical article. J Neurosurg 5:927–935. doi:10.3171/2009.4.JNS081649
12. Houkin K, Ishikawa T, Yoshimoto T, Abe H (1997) Direct and indirect revascularization for Moyamoya disease surgical techniques and peri-operative complications. Clin Neurol Neurosurg 99(Suppl 2):S142–S145
13. Janda V, Sachse J (2000) Manuelle Muskelfunktionsdiagnostik. 4. Auflage, Urban & Fischer.
14. Kawaguchi T, Fujita S, Hosoda K, Shose Y, Hamano S, Iwakura M et al (1996) Multiple burr-hole operation for adult Moyamoya disease. J Neurosurg 3:468–476. doi:10.3171/jns.1996.84.3.0468
15. Komotar RJ, Starke RM, Otten ML, Merkow MB, Garrett MC, Marshall RS et al (2009) The role of indirect extracranial-intracranial bypass in the treatment of symptomatic intracranial atheroocclusive disease. J Neurosurg 5:896–904. doi:10.3171/2008.9.JNS17658
16. Matsushima T, Inoue T, Ikezaki K, Matsukado K, Natori Y, Inamura T et al (1998) Multiple combined indirect procedure for the surgical treatment of children with Moyamoya disease. A comparison with single indirect anastomosis and direct anastomosis. Neurosurg Focus 5:e4
17. Matsushima T, Inoue T, Suzuki SO, Fujii K, Fukui M, Hasuo K (1992) Surgical treatment of moyamoya disease in pediatric

patients–comparison between the results of indirect and direct revascularization procedures. Neurosurgery 3:401–405
18. Mesiwala AH, Sviri G, Fatemi N, Britz GW, Newell DW (2008) Long-term outcome of superficial temporal artery-middle cerebral artery bypass for patients with Moyamoya disease in the US. Neurosurg Focus 2:E15. doi:10.3171/FOC/2008/24/2/E15
19. Reis CV, Safavi-Abbasi S, Zabramski JM, Gusmao SN, Spetzler RF, Preul MC (2006) The history of neurosurgical procedures for Moyamoya disease. Neurosurg Focus 6:E7
20. Scott RM, Smith ER (2009) Moyamoya disease and Moyamoya syndrome. N Engl J Med 12:1226–1237. doi:10.1056/NEJMra0804622
21. Smith ER, Scott RM (2005) Surgical management of Moyamoya syndrome. Skull Base 1:15–26. doi:10.1055/s-2005-868160
22. Starke RM, Komotar RJ, Connolly ES (2009) Optimal surgical treatment for moyamoya disease in adults: direct versus indirect bypass. Neurosurg Focus 4:E8. doi:10.3171/2009.01.FOCUS08309
23. Suzuki J, Takaku A (1969) Cerebrovascular "moyamoya" disease. Disease showing abnormal net-like vessels in base of brain. Arch Neurol 3:288–299
24. Takeuchi K, Shimizu K (1957) Hypoplasia of the bilateral internal carotid arteries. No To Shinkei 9:37–43
25. Wakai K, Tamakoshi A, Ikezaki K, Fukui M, Kawamura T, Aoki R et al (1997) Epidemiological features of Moyamoya disease in Japan: findings from a nationwide survey. Clin Neurol Neurosurg 99(Suppl 2):S1–S5
26. Yonekawa Y, Ogata N, Kaku Y, Taub E, Imhof HG (1997) Moyamoya disease in Europe, past and present status. Clin Neurol Neurosurg 99(Suppl 2):S58–S60. doi:10.1016/S0303-8467(97), 00042-5
27. Zipfel GJ, Fox DJJ, Rivet DJ (2005) Moyamoya disease in adults: the role of cerebral revascularization. Skull Base 1:27–41. doi:10.1055/s-2005-868161

7. Kim SK, Seol HJ, Cho BK, Hwang YS, Lee DS, Wang KC (2004) Moyamoya disease among young patients: its aggressive clinical course and the role of active surgical treatment. Neurosurgery 54:840–846
8. Matsushima T, Inoue T, Natori Y, Fujii K, Fukui M, Hasuo K, Kuwabara Y (1994) Children with unilateral occlusion or stenosis of the ICA associated with surrounding moyamoya vessels – "unilateral" Moyamoya disease. Acta Neurochir (Wien) 131:196–202
9. Scott RM, Smith ER (2009) Moyamoya disease and Moyamoya syndrome. N Engl J Med 360:1226–1237
10. Suzuki J, Takaku A (1969) Cerebrovascular "Moyamoya" disease: disease showing abnormal net-like vessel in base of brain. Arch Neurol 20:288–299
11. Yilmaz E, Pritz M, Bruno A, Lopez-Nunez A, Biller J (2001) Moyamoya: Indiana University Medical Center experience. Arch Neurol 58:1274–1278
12. Yonekawa Y, Ogata N, Kaku Y, Taub E, Imhof HG (1997) Moyamoya disease in Europe, past and present status. Clin Neurol Neurosurg 99(Suppl 2):558–560

Tissue Fusion, a New Opportunity for Sutureless Bypass Surgery

Serge Bogni, Daniel Schöni, Mihai Constantinescu, Amina Wirth, Istvan Vajtai, Amadé Bregy, Andreas Raabe, Uwe Pieles, Martin Frenz, and Michael Reinert

Abstract Microsurgical suturing is the standard for cerebral bypass surgery, a technique where temporary occlusion is usually necessary. Non-occlusive techniques such as excimer laser-assisted non-occlusive anastomosis (ELANA) have certainly widened the spectrum of treatment of complex cerebrovascular situations, such as giant cerebral aneurysms, that were otherwise non-treatable. Nevertheless, the reduction of surgical risks while widening the spectrum of indications, such as a prophylactic cerebral bypass, is still a main aim, that we would like to pursue with our sutureless tissue fusion research. The primary concern in sutureless tissue fusion- and especially in tissue fusion of cerebral vessels- is the lack of reproducibility, often caused by variations in the thermal damage of the vessel. This has prevented this novel fusion technique from being applicable in daily surgical use. In this overview, we present three ways to further improve the laser tissue soldering technique.

In the first section entitled "Laser Tissue Soldering Using a Biodegradable Polymer," a porous polymer scaffold doped with albumin (BSA) and indocyanine green (ICG) is presented, leading to strong and reproducible tensile strengths in tissue soldering. Histologies and future developments are discussed.

In the section "Numerical Simulation for Improvement of Laser Tissue Soldering," a powerful theoretical simulation model is used to calculate temperature distribution during soldering. The goal of this research is to have a tool in hand that allows us to determine laser irradiation parameters that guarantee strong vessel fusion without thermally damaging the inner structures such as the intima and endothelium.

In a third section, "Nanoparticles in Laser Tissue Soldering," we demonstrate that nanoparticles can be used to produce a stable and well-defined spatial absorption profile in the scaffold, which is an important step towards increasing the reproducibility. The risks of implanting nanoparticles into a biodegradable scaffold are discussed.

Step by step, these developments in sutureless tissue fusion have improved the tensile strength and the reproducibility, and are constantly evolving towards a clinically applicable anastomosis technique.

Introduction

The conventional technique for vascular tissue fusion is microsuturing. Suturing, however, has the inherent drawback of tissue perforation and of the possibility that suture material can lead to foreign body reactions, thrombocyte aggregation, impaired endothelial function, intimal hyperplasia and hence stenosis [18, 19, 26, 40, 41]. In addition, microsuturing not only requires specific surgical skills, but is often time consuming. This may be crucial in clinical conditions where temporary ischemia is an issue for the survival of the anastomosed tissue, such as the brain or after a transplant. Furthermore, suturing requires free moving space and is therefore only applicable with limitations for minimally invasive surgery.

Different techniques have been experimentally and clinically studied so far, such as micro-hole punchers and staplers for microanastomosis (Cardica) or non-occlusive anastomosis techniques such as excimer laser-assisted non-occlusive anastomosis (ELANA) [5, 10, 14, 16, 35]. The Cardica device has been shown to be applicable only on peripheral and superficial sites in the brain, and is accompanied by a

S. Bogni and M. Frenz
Institute of Applied Physics, University of Bern, Bern, Switzerland

D. Schöni A. Bregy, and A. Raabe
Department of Neurosurgery, Inselspital Bern, University of Bern, Bern, Switzerland

M. Constantinescu
Department of Plastic and Reconstructive Surgery, Inselspital Bern, University of Bern, Bern, Switzerland

A. Wirth and U. Pieles
Institute for Chemistry and Bioanalytics, Fachhochschule Nordwestschweiz, Basel, Switzerland

I. Vajtai
Institute of Pathology, University of Bern, Bern, Switzerland

M. Reinert (✉)
Institute of Applied Physics, University of Bern, Bern, Switzerland and
Department of Neurosurgery, Inselspital Bern, 3010, Bern, Switzerland
e-mail: mmv.reinert@insel.ch

T. Tsukahara et al. (eds.), *Trends in Neurovascular Surgery,* Acta Neurochirurgica Supplementum, Vol. 112,
DOI: 10.1007/978-3-7091-0661-7_9, © Springer-Verlag/Wien 2011

non-satisfying anastomosis patency rate and difficulties in handling. The ELANA technique has shown good clinical results, especially in the repair of the anterior brain circulation. However, it requires an expert team of surgeons and laser therapist, and thus is limited to a few centers.

Therefore, there is still a need for developing anastomosis techniques that can close these gaps. A possible solution could be sutureless laser tissue soldering (LTS) anastomosis since this technique is simple, fast and easy to perform, and can be applied to different vessel sizes and intraoperative locations both in open operations and endoscopically.

In LTS a chromophore-enhanced protein solder is put onto the anastomosis site, which absorbs the laser energy [7, 24, 25]. In most cases, bovine serum albumin (BSA) is used as a protein and indocyanine green (ICG) as a biocompatible chromophore. Direct heating of the solder and subsequently of the blood vessel wall by heat diffusion leads to denaturation of the solder and adjacent tissue, and thus to tissue fusion, which means that LTS is inherently connected to a certain amount of thermal tissue damage. Although the principle of LTS is not questioned, the molecular effects causing the acute connection strength are still controversially discussed [3, 9, 22]. Laser-soldered anastomoses form an immediate watertight connection. Furthermore, it has been shown that laser-soldered wounds have a better inflammatory response than sutured wounds [3, 33]. As the laser light can be delivered via optical fibers through a catheter, the anastomosis can be performed in a minimally invasive way [24, 27, 31]. Biodegradable polymers such as polyglycolic acid or polycaprolactone have been used as carrier material for the liquid solder. They prevent runaway of the liquid solder and give additional strength to the anastomosis [6, 15, 32, 33].

Different solder parameters, solder-surface temperatures and tissue response can be evaluated with in vitro and in vivo experiments. Such experiments, however, are costly and time consuming. Theoretical models can help to optimize the parameters as they allow us to calculate temperatures within the soldering site [8, 28, 29]. Thus, theoretical models can drastically reduce the number of experiments needed to optimize parameters for LTS. Previous work on LTS has shown that in order to obtain a strong tissue connection, solder temperatures exceeding 80°C are required, a temperature necessary to denaturate BSA [6, 13, 23]. In our theoretical model 80°C was therefore the target temperature for the solder/vessel contact layer (interface). Such a high temperature, however, can lead to severe vessel damage causing thrombosis, especially if the endothelium is damaged [12, 30, 37]. A difficulty in vascular LTS is to apply laser and solder parameters that allow high temperatures at the interface between the vessel wall and solder in order to guarantee a strong and liquid-tight fusion, but at the same time stay below the damage threshold of the endothelium. In a parameter study we therefore aimed at high temperature gradients (ΔT) within the vessel wall. Knowledge of the temperature field within the blood vessel and its temporal evolution is vital to understand the influence of device parameters and boundary conditions. LTS is inherently a coupled multiphysical problem where absorption of laser light, thermal diffusion and heat exchange with the surrounding environment need to be taken into account. Finite elements methods (FEM), such as the COMSOL Multiphysics program, are powerful tools to calculate temperature distributions.

In the following we describe different approaches and findings that improve the quality and reproducibility of sutureless vascular tissue fusion. First we describe the utility of using a biodegradable strong polymer host for the BSA and the light absorbing dye [6]. Secondly, we demonstrate how computer simulations can help to optimize the irradiation parameters to keep the thermal tissue damage as low as possible [4]. In the third part, we describe possible applications of nanoparticles used as selective absorbers to generate well-predefined and reproducible heat distribution inside the scaffold.

Laser Tissue Soldering Using a Biodegradable Polymer

One aim of this study was to optimize adhesion properties regarding reproducibility and tensile strength in tissue soldering of rabbit aortic arteries and to further improve our

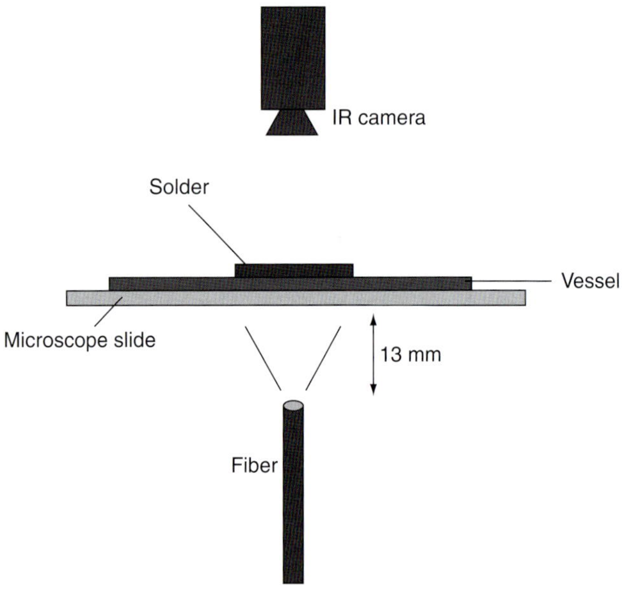

Fig. 1 Scheme of the soldering setup. A piece of aortic vessel was mounted with the adventitial side upward onto a microscope slide with the solder placed on top. Soldering was performed from the bottom through the aortic tissue using near-infrared diode laser ($\lambda = 808$ nm) radiation transmitted through a 400-μm core fiber. The spot size on the tissue bottom was 0.21 cm^2. During the soldering process, the solder surface temperature was recorded using an infrared camera. For details, see references Bregy et al. [6] and Bogni et al. [4]

intraluminal end-to-end soldering technique using a biodegradable polymer scaffold as a solder carrier material [24]. The experimental setup is shown in Fig. 1. All parameters such as laser irradiation, BSA concentration and its local distribution, tissue preparation and polymer scaffold production had been standardized to precisely determine their individual influence on the temperature distribution. The literature has shown that the use of a biodegradable polymer scaffold as carrier material helps to improve tensile strength in tissue soldering [32, 33]. In our study, we chose 5-mm-wide strips of polycaprolactone (PCL) as carrier material because of its low melting point at around 60°C [39]. The solder-soaked polymer scaffold was completely dried prior to use. We postulated that we could obtain a more homogenous and therefore stronger polymer–BSA–tissue interaction by melting the polymer at the interface. A further beneficial effect of the polymer scaffold is that different thicknesses or shapes such as tubes can be utilized to optimally adapt the scaffold to the surgical requirements.

The histologies (Fig. 2c1–c3) clearly show that the melted PCL creates a smooth seal at the interface between the scaffold and tissue, which we assume is an important factor for achieving good and reproducible tensile strengths. Our preliminary measurements ($n=3$) indicated that a higher energy deposition (either obtained by a high power or long irradiation times) resulted in stronger tissue bonds up to a maximum at which a further increase did not lead to higher tensile strengths (Fig. 3). This fact can be understood when analyzing the histologies. The stronger heating leads to an almost homogeneous intermixture of melted and denaturated BSA-doped scaffold and thermally coagulated vessel wall tissue. The homogeneous intermixture produced a high tensile strength,

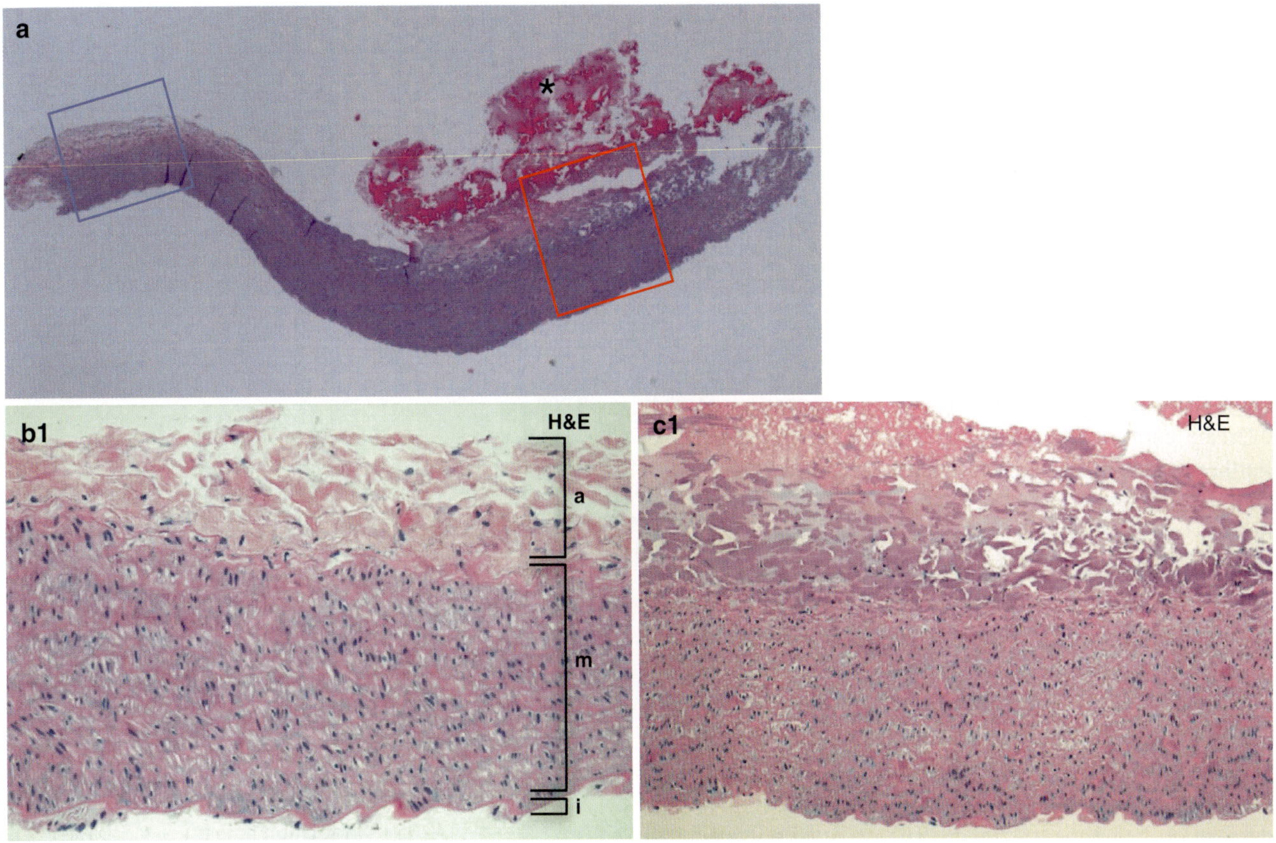

Fig. 2 Histology of vessel wall alterations locally induced by thermal effects of soldering at different soldering parameters. Histology is shown in H&E for assessment of cellular structural integrity. Van Gieson's elastic (EvG) is used for determination of the collagen matrix structure. A: Longitudinal whole-mount sections of rabbit aorta to show crust-like layer of coagulated soldering medium (*asterisk*) adherent to adventitia. *Blue* and *red boxes* indicate untreated control segment and soldered areas, respectively. (b1, B2) Detail view of native aortic wall architecture corresponding to the *blue box* in a. The intima (*i*) being rather nondescript, the thickness of this large artery is mostly comprised of a robust tunica media (*m*) replete with undulating elastic fibers, among which smooth muscle cells and fibroblasts are encased. Some of the elastic fibers along the outermost medial layer tend to gradually merge into the loose connective tissue of the adventitia (*a*). Note that interspersed nuclei of individual adventitial cells are clearly recognizable. (c1, c2): Using optimum soldering parameters (1.5 W and 60 s), thermal damage in the area soldered to the adventitia is evident (*red box in* a). In comparison to B1, most adventitial nuclei have disappeared, and collagen as well as elastic fibers tends to form a poorly structured amalgam. Conversely, the tunica media (i.e., the most dynamically relevant layer) appears largely unaffected by coagulative changes. A full set of morphologically intact nuclei is appreciated in c1. The intima is appreciated as intact in c1, c2. In c3 a higher magnification of c1, the melted BIP scaffold (*) creates a smooth seal of the tissue and scaffold at their interface. Overheating (using soldering parameters of 1.5 W and 240 s) tended to produce shrinkage (d1) and/or vacuolation (d2)

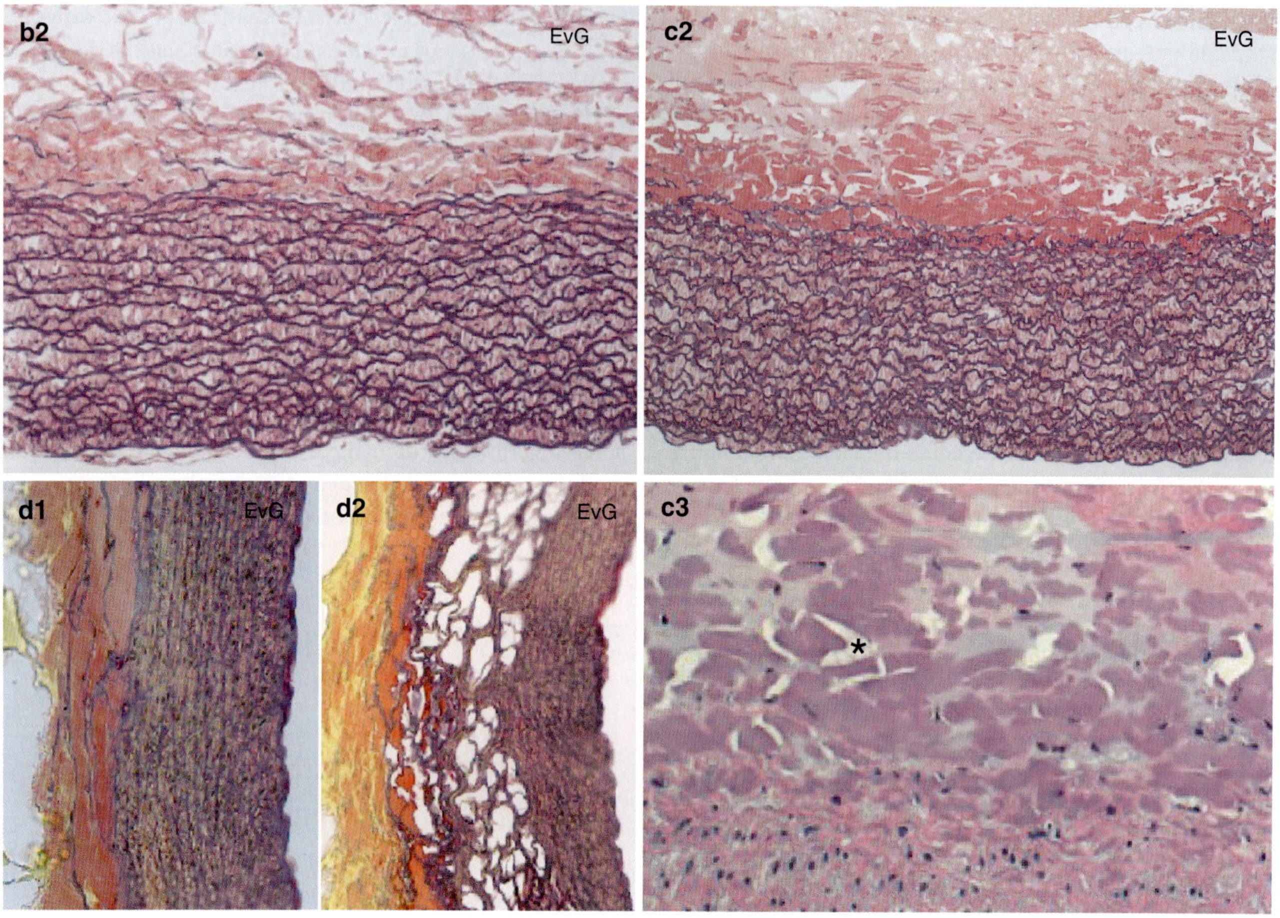

Fig. 2 (continued)

but at the expense of extensive tissue damage that can spread over the entire thickness of the vessel wall (Fig. 2d1, d2). Further increasing the temperature causes boiling of the tissue water, resulting in a pronounced shrinkage and/or appearance of vacuoles in the tissue. As a result, the maximum tensile strength obtained levels off or even decreases, as shown in Fig. 3. The comparison of laser power and irradiation time in combination with macroscopic and histological evaluation revealed that an irradiation power of 1.5 W with an irradiation time of 60 s, a clinically practicable time, was the optimal irradiation setting. The associated tissue damage was restricted to the adventitia and its interface with the outermost layer of the tunica media without evidence of dehydration (Fig. 2). No damage of the intima was found. The maximal polymer surface temperature was around 117°C. An ICG concentration of 1 mg/g was chosen to obtain the most homogenous absorption over the entire scaffold thickness.

The importance of a complete denaturation of the albumin to laser soldering is not well understood. However, in order to provide long-term wound closure and appropriate tensile strength, it seems to be very important that the solder is converted from a soluble to a non-soluble form. It is likely that this conversion occurs during the denaturation process, which is affected by many parameters. The effects of PCL and ICG on BSA denaturation have not yet been reported. However, it

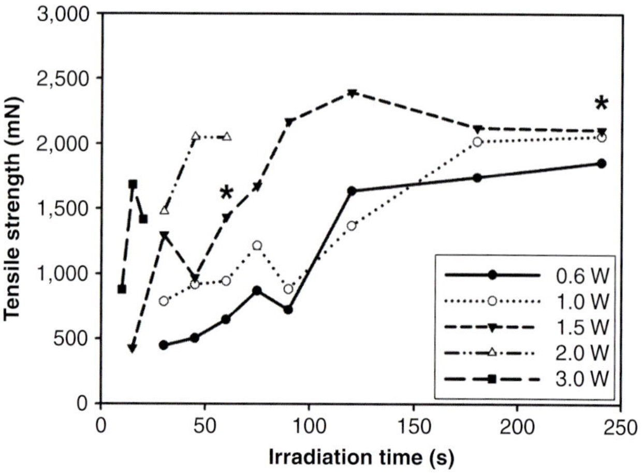

Fig. 3 Tensile strengths of soldered tissue vessels as a function of soldering time for different laser powers ($n \geq 3$ for each point). A higher energy deposition (either due to longer irradiation time or higher intensity) leads to a higher tensile strength. The two *asterisks* mark the irradiation parameters and resulting tensile strength of the soldered samples used for histology

has been reported that pH variations, purity grade and additives can change shape and temperature range of the BSA denaturation peak in differential scanning calorimetry (DSC) [1, 23, 38]. In a BSA polysaccharide system, Antonov and

Wolf have shown a shift of the denaturation peak towards lower temperatures with increasing polymer concentration [1]. An explanation is given that water structure is affected by the presence of the polymer, thus weakening the hydrophobic interactions in the tertiary structure of the protein. Moisture content affects protein denaturation accordingly, and this effect has long been observed and reported [2, 34]. The used solder scaffolds are dry when placed on the wound; however, the water content in the solder material increases with time because of water adsorption and diffusion. We therefore assume that BSA undergoes a complete first denaturation reaction everywhere in the scaffold. It is also likely that the second observed denaturation reaction occurs near the scaffold-tissue interface, where moisture content is supposed to be highest. This results in a gradient of the denaturation temperature over the thickness of the polymer scaffold, which strongly supports the soldering process. Cellular integrity during the soldering procedure, especially in the inner segments of the vessel, is the primary goal, which can be achieved by keeping the soldering temperature low. We could demonstrate that by increasing the moisture, the denaturation temperature can be reduced. Lowering the pH slightly, adding a hydrophilic substance or using a protein mixture such as albumin and globulin may further reduce the effective soldering temperature.

We and others have shown that increasing the BSA concentration results in stronger tensile strengths [17, 21]. We could show that the tensile strength became about 30% stronger (around 2,000±400 mN, which is about half of a native vessel) when increasing the BSA concentration from 25% to 40%. Since all the ruptures happened at the interface between the vessel wall and the scaffold, we can expect that the tensile strength of a soldered end-to-end vascular anastomosis could even be enlarged when increasing the contact area. As we have developed a promising tissue adhesion matrix, the next step will be to show the feasibility of this soldering procedure in vivo and to evaluate long-term effects of the soldering regarding healing strength and patency. Furthermore, knowledge of the developments described in the next two sections can be integrated into the production phase of the polymer scaffold.

Numerical Simulation for Improvement of Laser Tissue Soldering

Experimentally, only surface temperatures are accessible for non-contact temperature measurements. The quality of the tissue fusion, however, depends on the temperature at the interface between the vessel wall and solder scaffold and on the temperature at the intima as it determines the risk of stenosis [6, 12, 37]. A precise calculation of these temperatures helps to determine the optimum laser parameters and to reduce the number of experiments necessary to optimize the soldering technique.

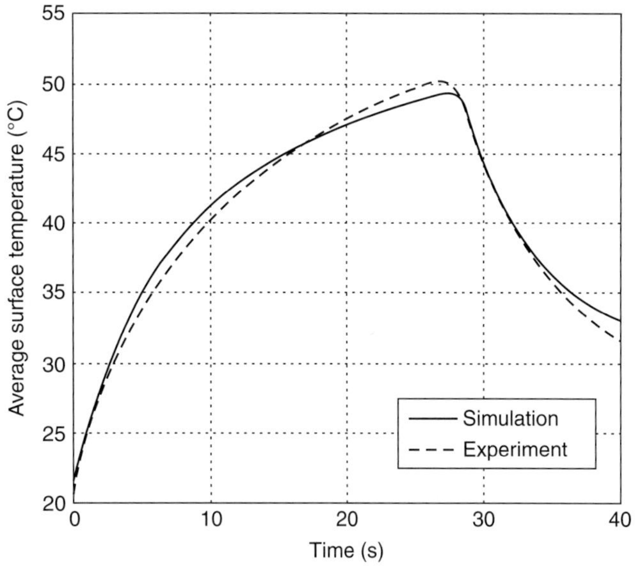

Fig. 4 Comparison of the solder surface temperature between simulation and experiment. Laser power 0.336-W solder absorption coefficient 192 cm^{-1}

We therefore aimed to develop a mathematical algorithm capable of determining the spatial and temporal temperature distribution inside the scaffold-tissue sample during the soldering process. The model was experimentally validated using the setup shown in Fig. 1. Our thermodynamic model calculates the time-resolved temperature distribution taking heat diffusion, convection and surface evaporation into account. Figure 4 shows an almost perfect agreement between the calculated and experimentally determined temperature development at the surface of the scaffold, which confirms the assumptions made and boundary conditions chosen in the simulation. The validated model can now be easily modified to describe in vivo conditions by adjusting the boundary conditions and material constants.

Previous experiments have revealed that for strong and tight soldering, the ICG-doped albumin scaffold needs to be heated at the interface to at least 80°C. Since the gradual process of irreversible BSA denaturation starts at around 70°C, heating to 80°C is also required to fully denaturate the albumin [13]. To avoid desiccation of the blood vessel and to keep soldering within a clinically acceptable time, we chose an irradiation time of maximum 30 s. To lower the risk of thrombosis after soldering, the intima temperature should stay as low as possible, but at least below its damage threshold [12, 37]. Therefore, a large temperature difference between the solder/vessel interface and intima (ΔT) was considered ideal. To evaluate the optimum parameter set, we varied the absorption properties of the solder, the laser power, irradiation mode (cw vs. pulsed), cooling of the lumen and the solder thickness over a wide parameter range. The highest absorption coefficient simulated was $\mu_a = 288$ cm^{-1}, the highest laser power 3 W. These values were chosen first because they were technically feasible, thus giving us

Table 1 Overview of the results for different laser powers

Laser power (W)	Absorption (cm^{-1})	Time in s	T interface	T intima	ΔT
3	192	2.5	88.4	60.7	27.7
1.52	192	6.55	82	66	16
1	192	14.1	80.2	70	10.2
0.8	192	24.7	80.3	72.6	7.7
0.8	288	19.7	80.2	71.6	8.6
3	288	2	84.9	56.2	28.5

T in °C. Simulations that did not reach an interface temperature of 80°C within the required 30 s are not displayed

the possibility to compare the experiment and simulation. Secondly, if further increasing the absorption coefficient, the energy is deposited in a very thin solder layer. An absorption coefficient of 288 cm^{-1} already results in an optical penetration depth of only 35 μm. Since heating of the solder scaffold is the result of heat diffusion, the polymer can only be denaturated over its entire thickness when using longer irradiation times. This however causes severe intimal damage. The parameter study showed that the combination of a high solder absorption ($\mu_a = 288$ cm^{-1}), a laser power of 3 W and an irradiation time of only a few seconds results in a steep temperature gradient within the vessel wall (Table 1). On the other hand, it is well known that protein and tissue denaturation follows an Arrhenius type rate process. Therefore, it is not only the temperature, but also the time-temperature history that describes denaturation. A single pulse that generates an interface temperature of 80°C may not be sufficient to fully denaturate the solder. The solution to this problem is a repetitively pulsed irradiation. Pulsed energy deposition can lead to ΔT values of over 30 K even if the mean energy deposition is the same as in continuous irradiation, where ΔT is below 16 K (Fig. 5). A pulsed irradiation therefore seems to better fulfill our initial requirements.

Figure 5 shows a temperature increase at the interface above 100°C. This leads to water evaporation inside the tissue causing vacuolization, which strongly changes the mechanical and thermal properties [6, 20, 25]. Vacuolization lowers the heat diffusion, resulting in a slower cooling of the sample. Such changes in thermal material properties during the soldering procedure are not considered in our simulations. Furthermore, vacuolization leads to a decrease in tensile strength of the blood vessel and therefore of the anastomosis [6]. Since high laser powers and high absorption coefficients lead to high ΔT values, vacuolization should be avoided by reducing the pulse duration.

During the simulations we also varied the solder thickness. This factor has however only a minor impact on ΔT. Even though we expect a thicker solder layer to provide additional stability to the anastomosis, it does not seem to be an optimal setting as lowering of the temperature leads to longer irradiation times and therefore higher risk of tissue damage. In order to overcome this drawback, changes in the composition of the solder scaffold, such as decreasing porosity or combining different polymers, is the next step to be studied.

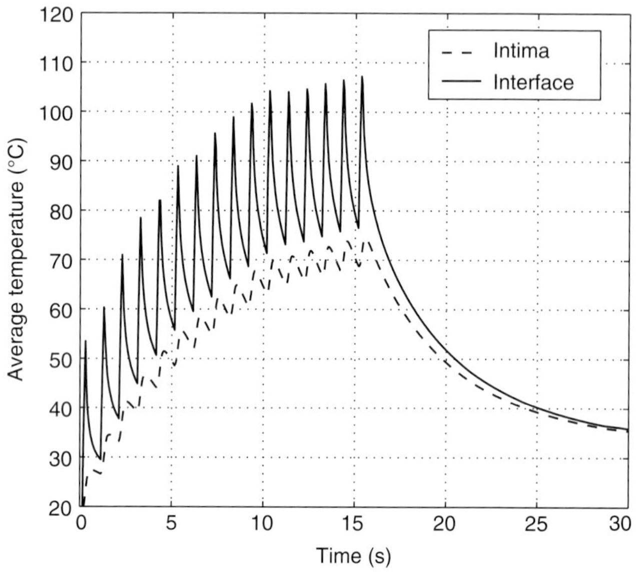

Fig. 5 Comparison between intima and interface temperature. Laser operating in pulsed mode at 1 Hz, 30% duty cycle with average power of 1.52 W. Solder absorption coefficient $\mu_a = 192$ cm^{-1}

Efficient cooling of the lumen would be another way to prevent damage of the intima. A temperature gradient of 54 K could be reached within the vessel wall if keeping the temperature in the vessel lumen constant at 30°C.

The simulations revealed that optimum soldering results are obtained when short pulsed irradiation with a high laser power and a highly absorbing solder is used. If the pulse duration is adjusted such that it fulfills the condition of thermal confinement, which means that the heat does not diffuse during its deposition, high temperature gradients within the vessel wall can be realized. Figure 6 shows an example in which the solder/vessel interface was repetitively heated above 80°C, while the intima temperature stayed below 65°C.

Nanoparticles in Laser Tissue Soldering

A remarkable improvement in view of reproducibility was the use of a polymer host for the BSA and the absorbing dye since it prevented the solder from running away during the soldering process. Unfortunately, the ICG passively taken up by the polymer scaffold is still water soluble, meaning that in an aqueous

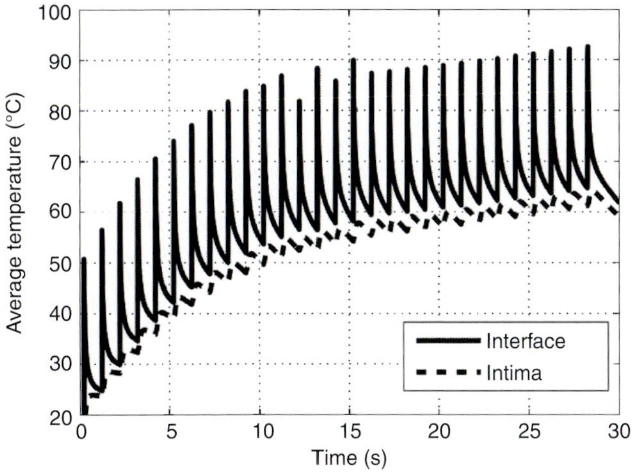

Fig. 6 Comparison between intima and interface temperature. Laser operating in pulsed mode at 1 Hz, 0.6% duty cycle with average power of 0.3 W. Solder absorption coefficient $\mu_a = 288\ cm^{-1}$

in vivo situation the absorbing ICG dilutes, leading again to a non-reproducible temperature increase within the soldering site and therefore to strong variations in the soldered strength. To overcome this drawback, the dye has to be actively bound to the polymer, which can be done using nanotechnology.

Core shell silica nanoparticles (250–270 nm in diameter) containing the ICG dye can be directly bound to the polymer scaffold. The dye encapsulation eliminates natural dye diffusion and thus allows us to produce almost any spatial absorber distribution inside the polymer to optimize the thermal response.

The nanoshells are conveniently prepared by a water-in-oil microemulsion or by Stoeber methods [11]. Using this water-in-oil approach, the aqueous phase will be used to entrap and immobilize active species [36]. Owing to this high versatility, we use fully characterized core shell silica nanoparticles for encapsulation. With regard to the preparation of the silica-encapsulated form of ICG, the synthetic approach is divided into three different phases (Fig. 7):

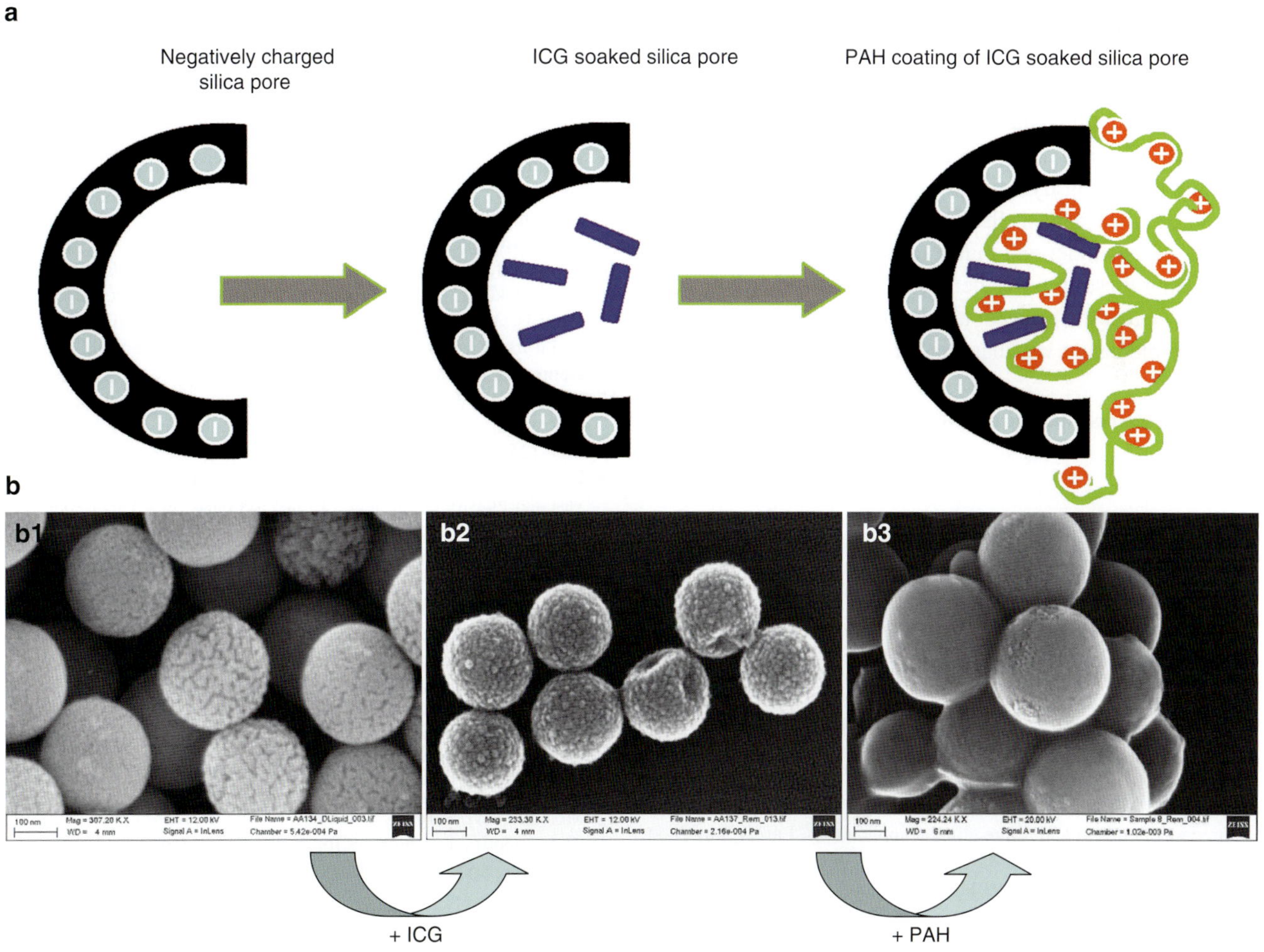

Fig. 7 (**a**) Schematic illustration of the surface coating of mesoporous silica particles encapsulating ICG with polyallylamine hydrochloride. (**b**) Field emission scanning electron microscope (FE SEM) micrographs of mesoporous silica particles (i) before addition of ICG dye, (ii) after incorporation of ICG dye, (iii) after surface coating of the particles with PAH polymer

Phase 1: synthesis of mesoporous silica nanoparticles in the form of nanoshells with tunable size and porosity.

Phase 2: incorporation of a substantial amount of ICG into the silica nanoshells.

Phase 3: wrapping/coating the surface of the so-encapsulated ICG into silica with poly (allylamine hydrochloride), a cationic polyelectrolyte, which adsorbs electrostatically to the negatively charged silica surface.

These nanoshells bind to the polymer scaffold using the normal solvent casting and particulate leaching technique also described in Bregy et al. [6].

However, the effect of these nanoshells in view of toxicity and biodistribution has to be carefully studied before such modified scaffolds can be used clinically.

Conclusion

Laser tissue fusion has been evolving over the last five decades from simply coagulating pieces of tissue together to a more sophisticated technique using additional protein solders, chromophores and solder carrier materials. In a first study we introduced a polymer (polycaprolactone) scaffold as a promising solder carrier material. In the second section we presented the prospects of a numerical model as an additional tool to optimize laser settings and optical properties of the solder. The last section presents a technique for how to bind the absorbing dye directly to the polymer scaffold by the aid of silica nanoshells. This guarantees a reproducible heating of the solder and thus a reproducible tissue connection. Using these improvements we progressed from (occasionally successful) anecdotal end-to-end tissue fusion to reproducible patent vascular anastomosis.

Conflict of interest statement We declare that we have no conflict of interest.

References

1. Antonov YA, Wolf BA (2005) Calorimetric and structural investigation of the interaction between bovine serum albumin and high molecular weight dextran in water. Biomacromolecules 6(6): 2980–2989
2. Barker HA (1933) The effect of water content upon the rate of heat denaturation of crystallizable egg albumin. J Gen Physiol 17(1): 21–34
3. Bass LS, Treat MR (1995) Laser tissue welding: a comprehensive review of current and future clinical applications. Lasers Surg Med 17(4):315–349
4. Bogni S, Stumpp O, Reinert M, Frenz M (2010) Thermal model for optimization of vascular laser tissue soldering. J Biophotonics 3(5–6):284–295
5. Bregy A, Alfieri A, Demertzis S, Mordasini P, Jetzer AK, Kuhlen D, Schaffner T, Dacey R, Steiger H-J, Reinert M (2008) Automated end-to-side anastomosis to the middle cerebral artery: a feasibility study. J Neurosurg 108(3):567–574
6. Bregy A, Bogni S, Bernau VJP, Vajtai I, Vollbach F, Petri-Fink A, Constantinescu M, Hofmann H, Frenz M, Reinert M (2008) Solder doped polycaprolactone scaffold enables reproducible laser tissue soldering. Lasers Surg Med 40(10):716–725
7. Byrd BD, Heintzelman DL, McNally-Heintzelman KM (2003) Absorption properties of alternative chromophores for use in laser tissue soldering applications. Biomed Sci Instrum 39:6–11
8. Cain CP, Polhamus GD, Roach WP, Stolarski DJ, Schuster KJ, Stockton KL, Rockwell BA, Chen B, Welch AJ (2006) Porcine skin visible lesion thresholds for near-infrared lasers including modeling at two pulse durations and spot sizes. J Biomed Opt 11(4):041109
9. Constantinescu MA, Alfieri A, Mihalache G, Stuker F, Ducray A, Seiler RW, Frenz M, Reinert M (2007) Effect of laser soldering irradiation on covalent bonds of pure collagen. Lasers Med Sci 22(1):10–14
10. Dacey RG, Zipfel GJ, Ashley WW, Chicoine MR, Reinert M (2008) Automated, compliant, high-flow common carotid to middle cerebral artery bypass. J Neurosurg 109(3):559–564
11. Ekwall P, Mandell L, Fontell K (1970) Some observations on binary and ternary aerosol OT systems. J Colloid Interface Sci 33(2):215–235
12. Fajardo LF, Schreiber AB, Kelly NI, Hahn GM (1985) Thermal sensitivity of endothelial cells. Radiat Res 103(2):276–285
13. Farahnaky A, Badii F, Farhat IA, Mitchell JR, Hill SE (2005) Enthalpy relaxation of bovine serum albumin and implications for its storage in the glassy state. Biopolymers 78(2):69–77
14. Hänggi D, Reinert M, Steiger H-J (2009) C Port Flex A assisted automated anastomosis high flow extracranial intracranial bypass surgery patients symptomatic carotid artery occlusion feasibility study. Clinical article. J Neurosurg 111(1):181–187
15. Hoffman GT, Soller EC, McNally-Heintzelman KM (2002) Biodegradable synthetic polymer scaffolds for reinforcement of albumin protein solders used for laser-assisted tissue repair. Biomed Sci Instrum 38:53–58
16. Langer DJ, Van Der Zwan A, Vajkoczy P, Kivipelto L, Van Doormaal TP, Tulleken CA (2008) Excimer laser-assisted nonocclusive anastomosis. An emerging technology for use in the creation of intracranial-intracranial and extracranial-intracranial cerebral bypass. Neurosurg Focus 24(2):E6
17. Lauto A (1998) Repair strength dependence on solder protein concentration: a study in laser tissue-welding. Lasers Surg Med 22(2): 120–125
18. Lidman D, Daniel RK (1981) The normal healing process of microvascular anastomoses. Scand J Plast Reconstr Surg 15(2):103–110
19. Macchiarelli G, Familiari G, Caggiati A, Magliocca FM, Riccardelli F, Miani A, Motta PM (1991) Arterial repair after microvascular anastomosis. Scanning and transmission electron microscopy study. Acta Anat 140(1):8–16
20. Mausberg R, Visser H, Aschoff T, Donath K, Krüger W (1993) Histology of laser- and high-frequency-electrosurgical incisions in the palate of pigs. J Craniomaxillofac Surg 21(3):130–132
21. McNally KM, Sorg BS, Chan EK, Welch AJ, Dawes JM, Owen ER (1999) Optimal parameters for laser tissue soldering. Part I: tensile strength scanning electron microscopy analysis. Lasers Surg Med 24(5):319–331
22. McNally KM, Sorg BS, Chan EK, Welch AJ, Dawes JM, Owen ER (2000) Optimal parameters for laser tissue soldering: II. Premixed versus separate dye solder techniques. Lasers Surg Med 26(4): 346–356
23. Michnik A (2002) Thermal stability of bovine serum albumin DSC study. J Therm Anal Calorim 71(2):509–519

24. Ott B, Constantinescu MA, Erni D, Banic A, Schaffner T, Frenz M (2004) Intraluminal laser light source and external solder: in vivo evaluation of a new technique for microvascular anastomosis. Lasers Surg Med 35(4):312–316
25. Ott B, Züger BJ, Erni D, Banic A, Schaffner T, Weber HP, Frenz M (2001) Comparative in vitro study of tissue welding using a 808 nm diode laser and a Ho:YAG laser. Lasers Med Sci 16(4):260–266
26. Pagnanelli DM, Pait TG, Rizzoli HV, Kobrine AI (1980) Scanning electron micrographic study of vascular lesions caused by microvascular needles and suture. J Neurosurg 53(1):32–36
27. Poppas D, Sutaria P, Sosa RE, Mininberg D, Schlossberg S (1993) Chromophore enhanced laser welding of canine ureters in vitro using a human protein solder: a preliminary step for laparoscopic tissue welding. J Urol 150(3):1052–1055
28. Ratto F, Matteini P, Rossi F, Menabuoni L, Tiwari N, Kulkarni SK, Pini R (2009) Photothermal effects in connective tissues mediated by laser-activated gold nanorods. Nanomedicine 5(2):143–151
29. Rossi F, Pini R, Menabuoni L (2007) Experimental and model analysis on the temperature dynamics during diode laser welding of the cornea. J Biomed Opt 12(1):014031
30. Sahu SK, Song CW (1991) Thermal sensitivity and kinetics of thermotolerance in bovine aortic endothelial cells in culture. Int J Hyperthermia 7(1):103–111
31. Shumalinsky D, Lobik L, Cytron S, Halpern M, Vasilyev T, Ravid A, Katzir A (2004) Laparoscopic laser soldering for repair of ureteropelvic junction obstruction in the porcine model. J Endourol 18(2):177–181
32. Sorg BS, Welch AJ (2001) Laser-tissue soldering with biodegradable polymer films in vitro: film surface morphology and hydration effects. Lasers Surg Med 28(4):297–306
33. Sorg BS, Welch AJ (2003) Preliminary biocompatibility experiment of polymer films for laser-assisted tissue welding. Lasers Surg Med 32(3):215–223
34. Tsukada H, Takano K, Hattori M, Yoshida T, Kanuma S, Takahashi K (2006) Effect of sorbed water on the thermal stability of soybean protein. Biosci Biotechnol Biochem 70(9):2096–2103
35. van Doormaal TP, van der Zwan A, Verweij BH, Han KS, Langer DJ, Tulleken CA (2008) Treatment of giant middle cerebral artery aneurysms with a flow replacement bypass using the excimer laser-assisted nonocclusive anastomosis technique. Neurosurgery 63(1): 12–20, discussion 20–12
36. Wang F-C, Yuan R, Chai Y-Q (2006) Direct electrochemical immunoassay based on a silica nanoparticles/sol-gel composite architecture for encapsulation of immunoconjugate. Appl Microbiol Biotechnol 72(4):671–675
37. Ward PA, Till GO (1990) Pathophysiologic events related to thermal injury of skin. J Trauma 30(12 Suppl):S75–S79
38. Yamasaki M, Yano H, Aoki K (1990) Differential scanning calorimetric studies on bovine serum albumin: I. Effects of pH and ionic strength. Int J Biol Macromol 12(4):263–268
39. Yang S, Leong KF, Du Z, Chua CK (2001) The design of scaffolds for use in tissue engineering. Part I. Traditional factors. Tissue Eng 7(6):679–689
40. Zeebregts CJ, Heijmen RH, van den Dungen JJ, van Schilfgaarde R (2003) Non-suture methods of vascular anastomosis. Br J Surg 90(3):261–271
41. Zeebregts C, van den Dungen J, Buikema H, van der Want J, van Schilfgaarde R (2001) Preservation of endothelial integrity and function in experimental vascular anastomosis with non-penetrating clips. Br J Surg 88(9):1201–1208

STA-MCA Bypass for the Treatment of Ischemic Stroke

Kenji Kanamaru, Tomohiro Araki, Fumihiro Kawakita, Kazuhide Hamada, Hideki Kanamaru, Keita Matsuura, Akitoshi Sato, and Hidenori Suzuki

Abstract It is considered controversial whether superficial temporal artery (STA)-middle cerebral artery (MCA) bypass affects the outcome of patients with ischemic stroke. This prospective study was undertaken to demonstrate the effect of STA-MCA bypass on the cerebral blood flow and neurological status of the patients with ischemic stroke. Seventy-five patients underwent unilateral or bilateral STA-MCA bypass surgery. The selection of the patients closely adhered to the criteria of the Japan EC-IC Bypass Trial (JET). Cerebral blood flow (CBF) before and after Diamox administration was measured by single photon emission computed tomography (SPECT) using iodine-123-*N*-isopropyl-*p*-iodo-amphetamine (IMP). MRI, contrast-enhanced 3D CT scans, and angiography were performed on each patient pre- and postoperatively. Bypass surgery was successfully done in all patients. CBF was significantly increased after STA-MCA bypass ($P<0.05$). In addition, reservation of CBF was significantly improved after STA-MCA bypass ($P<0.05$). Patients with transient ischemic attack (TIA) did not experience recurrence of such episodes after STA-MCA bypass. The neurological deficit was unchanged in patients with complete stroke after bypass surgery. However, the NIH stroke scale was significantly improved after bypass surgery ($P<0.01$). In addition, the satisfaction rate of treatment as assessed by the patients themselves was very high after STA-MCA bypass (>90%) compared to the conservative treatment group (<50%). STA-MCA bypass still plays a limited role in the treatment of ischemic stroke, but may become a bright hope in depressed patients after cerebral ischemia.

Keywords Ischemic stroke · STA-MCA bypass · CBF · Cerebrovascular reservation capacity · NIH stroke scale

Introduction

Although attractive from a conceptual point of view, in an international randomized trial extracranial (EC)-intracranial (IC) artery bypass surgery was shown to be ineffective in preventing stroke [1]. However, some pilot studies demonstrated that cerebrovascular reserve capacity significantly improved over time after bypass [5]. Also, after bypass surgery, the mean regional cerebral blood flow (rCBF) value on the affected side was increased significantly, and the mean regional oxygen extraction fraction (rOEF) value on the affected side was significantly decreased [4]. Recently, the guideline for EC-IC bypass was published in Japan [6]. The indication for EC-IC bypass is as follows: (1) cases with TIA or minor stroke within 3 months of ictus in the age range under 73 years presenting with modified Rankin Scale score of 1 or 2; (2) no extensive infarction in the territory of large arteries on either CT scans or MRI with severe stenosis or occlusion of ICA or proximal MCA on cerebral angiograms; and (3) rCBF is under 80% of normal range and cerebrovascular reserve capacity is under 10% in the territory of the MCA using single-photon emission tomography (SPECT) or cold xenon CT at least 3 weeks after the latest attack [6]. Therefore, we prospectively collected 75 cases of ischemic stroke that met the criteria of EC-IC bypass as mentioned above and demonstrated an improvement both in rCBF and NIH stroke scale after EC-IC bypass.

K. Kanamaru (✉), T. Araki, F. Kawakita, K. Hamada, and H. Kanamaru
Department of Neurosurgery, Suzuka Kaisei Hospital, Suzuka, Japan and
Department of Neurology, Suzuka Kaisei Hospital, Suzuka, Japan
e-mail: kanamaru@h6.dion.ne.jp

A. Sato
Rehabilitation, Suzuka Kaisei Hospital, Suzuka, Japan

H. Suzuki
Department of Neurosurgery, Mie University School of Medicine, Tsu, Japan

T. Tsukahara et al. (eds.), *Trends in Neurovascular Surgery*, Acta Neurochirurgica Supplementum, Vol. 112,
DOI: 10.1007/978-3-7091-0661-7_10, © Springer-Verlag/Wien 2011

Table 1 Arterial lesion of the patients

ICA stenosis	11
ICA occlusion	24
MCA stenosis	17
MCA occlusion	16
Bilateral ICA stenosis	4
Moyamoya disease	3

Materials and Methods

Between 2000 and 2010, we treated 75 patients with STA-MCA bypass at Suzuka Kaisei Hospital, of whom 57 were men and 18 women, ranging in age from 28 to 81 years (mean, 64 years). Preoperative diagnoses are listed in Table 1. All patients underwent diagnostic studies, including MRI, cerebral angiograms, and measurement of rCBF. Pre- and postoperative studies of rCBF were performed in 30 patients using iodine-123-*N*-isopropyl-*p*-iodoamphetamine (IMP) SPECT [3]. Antiplatelet drugs were not stopped during the perioperative period. Single or double STA-MCA anastomosis was performed in all cases on the side of the compromised rCBF. Following a linear skin incision of the temporal muscle, a craniectomy of approximately 3 cm in diameter was made over the temporoparietal junction. This overlies the posterior sylvian fissure and provides access to suitably sized proximal cortical branches of the MCA as they rise. Donor and recipient arteries were anastomosed with interrupted 10-0 sutures under the operating microscope. The NIH stroke scale was measured, and the satisfaction rate was obtained from all patients pre- and postoperatively by the occupational therapist (AS), who was unaware of the history of surgery. Statistical evaluation of the results was carried out using the paired *t*-test. A value of $P < 0.05$ indicated a significant difference.

Results

Two patients died suddenly of myocardial infarction 2 weeks postoperatively after an initially uneventful postoperative course (2.7%). There were no other postoperative complications. No patient experienced a recurrence of ischemic attack postoperatively. Postoperative follow-up studies of cerebrovascular reserve capacity showed a significant increase over the operated side 1 month after surgery (Fig. 1). Remarkably, the NIH stroke scale was significantly improved postoperatively (Fig. 2). It is inferred that STA-MCA bypass is effective not only for the prevention of ischemic attack, but also for improvement of neurological function. The impressive satisfaction rate, taken from patients at discharge, was over 90%.

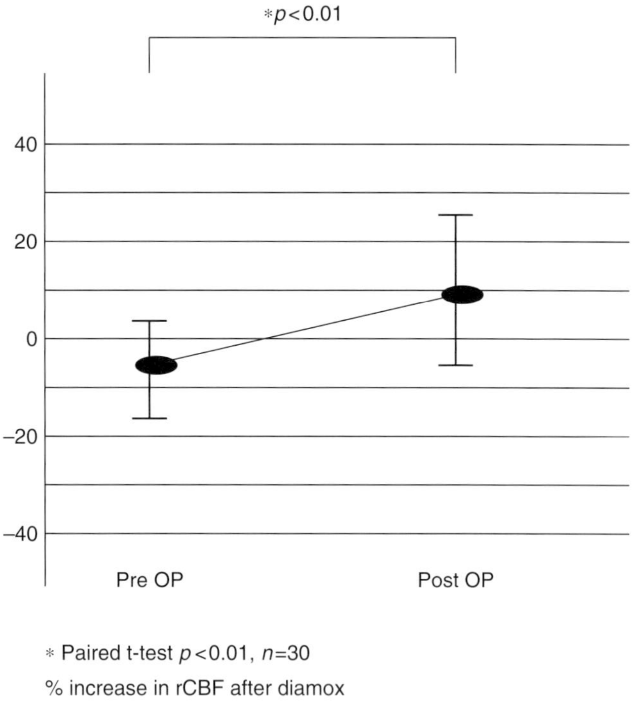

Fig. 1 Changes in cerebrovascular reserve capacity pre- and postoperatively

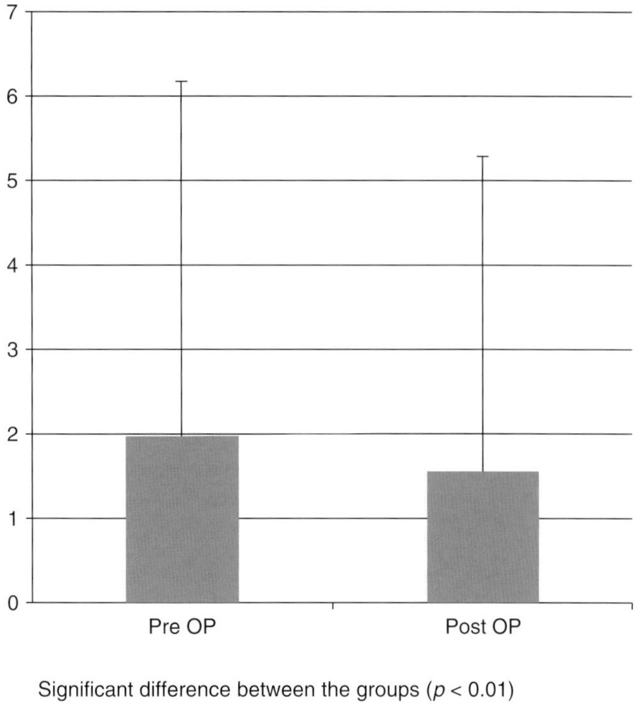

Fig. 2 Changes in NIH stroke score pre- and postoperatively

Discussion

In a series of 39 patients with hemodynamic compromise shown by the high oxygen extraction fraction on PET, the 2-year rate of ipsilateral ischemic stroke was 26.5% [2]. It is a recognized clinical dilemma that the patients who in theory have the most to gain from EC/IC bypass surgery also carry the highest perioperative risk [7]. One study reported a complication rate of conventional STA-MCA bypass surgery close to 12% in patients considered neurologically unstable [7]. Another study found a complication rate of 14% (major morbidity or death in 4 of 28 patients) of the conventional STA-MCA operation in patients with unilateral ICA occlusion who had recurrent symptoms and were hemodynamically compromised on the basis of 133Xe-SPECT measurements before and after acetazolamide challenge [5]. No postoperative ischemic complications were noted in our series. One reason may be that an antiplatelet drug was continued from admission to discharge, even in the perioperative period. Our complication rate (mortality rate = 2.7%) seems remarkably low. As in many other reports, cerebrovascular reserve capacity significantly improved after STA-MCA bypass in the present study [4, 5]. However, few reports have demonstrated neurological improvement after STA-MCA bypass. Our study showed that the NIH stroke scale was significantly improved after STA-MCA bypass. Our results need to be interpreted as follows: (1) we have been running the stroke center for 10 years, and multidisciplinary treatment of ischemic stroke has been established; (2) postoperative rehabilitation continued at least 1 year after STA-MCA bypass; and (3) the main operating surgeons (KK, TA) are responsible for observing their own patients from the hospital to the outpatient clinic, and this may comfort the patients.

In conclusion, our preliminary data are encouraging, and neurological improvement after STA-MCA bypass warrants further investigation.

Conflict of interest statement We declare that we have no conflict of interest.

References

1. The EC/IC Bypass Study Group (1985) Failure of extracranial-intracranial arterial bypass to reduce the risk of ischemic stroke. Results international randomized trial. N Engl J Med 313: 1191–1200
2. Grubb RL Jr, Derdeyn CP, Fritsch SM, Carpenter DA, Yundt KD, Videen TO, Spitznagel EL, Powers WJ (1998) Importance of hemodynamic factors in the prognosis of symptomatic carotid occlusion. JAMA 280:1055–1060
3. Iida H, Itoh H, Nakazawa M, Hatazawa J, Nishimura H, Onishi Y, Uemura K (1994) Quantitative mapping of regional cerebral blood flow using iodine-123-IMP and SPECT. J Nucl Med 35: 2019–2030
4. Iwama T, Hashimoto N, Hayashi K (2001) Cerebral hemodynamic parameters for patients with neurological improvements after extracranial-intracranial arterial bypass surgery: evaluation using positron emission tomography. Neurosurgery 48:504–512
5. Schmiedek P, Piepgras A, Leisinger G, Kirsche CM, Einhaupl K (1994) Improvement of cerebrovascular reserve capacity by EC-IC arterial bypass surgery in patients with ICA occlusion and hemodynamic cerebral ischemia. J Neurosurg 81:236–244
6. Shinohara Y (2009) 4-10. EC-IC Bypass. In: Shinohara Y, Ogawa A, Suzuki N, Katayama Y, Kimura A (eds) Japanese guidelines for the management of stroke 2009. Kyowa Kikaku, Tokyo, pp 126–127
7. Sundt TM, Whisnant JP, Fode NC, Piepgrass DG, Houser OW (1985) Results, complications, and follow-up of 415 bypass operations for occlusive disease of the carotid system. Mayo Clin Proc 60:230–240

The New MRI Modalities "BPAS and VISTA" for the Diagnosis of VA Dissection

Koichiro Takemoto, Koichi Takano, Hiroshi Abe, Masakazu Okawa, Mitsutoshi Iwaasa, Toshio Higashi, and Tooru Inoue

Abstract *Objective*: Recently VA dissection has drawn attention as a relatively common cause of stroke because of the introduction of MRI as a diagnostic technique. Basiparallel anatomic scanning (BPAS) was designed to visualize the surface appearance of the vertebrobasilar artery within the cistern. Volumetric isotropic TSE acquisition (VISTA) is a sort of black blood imaging method to evaluate the arterial wall and lumen. In this study, we aimed to evaluate the efficacy of the new MRI modalities "BPAS and VISTA," and to present a retrospective analysis of our experience with the diagnosis.

Materials and *methods*: Between1995 and 2010, we experienced 24 cases of VA dissection at our institution. In our cases, we could obtain images of 15 in BPAS and VISTA in addition to MRA. The mean age of the 15 patients (12 male and 3 female) was 51 years old (range 18–80). Ten of fifteen patients presented with ischemia, and 5/15 with only headache. There were no cases of SAH. In BPAS, we evaluated dilatation of the external diameter of the affected artery. We compared the findings in BPAS with MRA to evaluate the discrepancy. In VISTA, we evaluated its capability to distinguish intramural hematoma.

Result: Thirteen of fifteen patients presented with dilatation of the external diameter on BPAS. By comparing the findings in BPAS with MRA, we found a discrepancy in 8/15 cases (53%). We could detect intramural hematoma by using VISTA in 9/15 cases (60%). Thirteen of fifteen patients received follow-up MRI. Temporal change of the arterial shape was confirmed in 7/13 cases (53.8%).

Conclusion: Dilatation of the external diameter was shown highly frequently in VA dissections. In addition, a discrepancy between BPAS and MRA as well as the intramural hematoma on VISTA was found comparatively frequently. BPAS and VISTA are minimally invasive and useful methods as screening tests.

Keywords Vertebral artery dissection · BPAS · VISTA

Introduction

VA dissection has recently drawn attention as a relatively common cause of stroke because of the introduction of MRI as a diagnostic technique. In neuroimaging of dissections, confirming the arterial lumen abnormality was the old standard. Subsequently intramural hematoma was recognized as the definitive finding [3, 5, 6]. In recent reports, much attention has been paid to the surface appearance of the affected artery. According to the SCADS (Spontaneous Cervicocephalic Arterial Dissections Study) Japan criteria, in addition to findings of the arterial lumen and its temporal changes, detecting dilatation of the external diameter combined with narrowing or occlusion of the arterial lumen enabled to make the diagnosis of dissection. Recently, we have often used the new MRI modalities "BPAS and VISTA" for the diagnosis of VA dissection. BPAS is a simple MR imaging technique to visualize the surface appearance of the vertebrobasilar artery within the cistern. It is useful to judge the condition of the artery, whether it is dilatation, normal or hypoplasia. VISTA is a sort of black blood imaging method. It is effective to evaluate the arterial wall and lumen. In this study, we aimed to evaluate the efficacy of the new MRI modalities "BPAS and VISTA," and to present a retrospective analysis of our experience in the diagnosis.

Material and Methods

Between 1995 and 2010, we experienced 24 cases of VA dissection at Fukuoka University Hospital. The diagnosis of VA dissection was made based on characteristic features,

K. Takemoto (✉), H. Abe, M. Okawa, M. Iwaasa,
T. Higashi, and T. Inoue
Department of Neurosurgery, Fukuoka University School of Medicine, 7-45-1 Nanakuma, Jounan-ku, Fukuoka-shi, 814-0180 Fukuoka, Japan
e-mail: take9016@fukuoka-u.ac.jp

K. Takano
Department of Radiology, Fukuoka University School of Medicine, Fukuoka, Japan

DOI: 10.1007/978-3-7091-0661-7_11,

which were demonstrated on both the conventional angiography and MRI (pearl-and-string sign, string sign, tapered occlusion, intimal flap and intramural hematoma on T1-weighted image, dilatation of the extra-diameter on BPAS). In the 24 patients, we could obtain the images of 15 on conventional angiography, BPAS and VISTA in addition to MRA. In BPAS, we evaluated dilatation of the external diameter on the affected artery. We compared the findings in BPAS with MRA to evaluate the discrepancy. In VISTA, we evaluated its capability to distinguish intramural hematoma.

Patient Population

In our cases, we could obtain the images of 15 patients in BPAS and VISTA in addition to MRA. The mean age of the 15 patients (12 male and 3 female) was 51 years old (range 18–80). Ten of fifteen patients presented with ischemia, and 5/15 with only headache. There were no cases of SAH. In 9 patients, the initial MRI was performed within 2 weeks after the onsets.

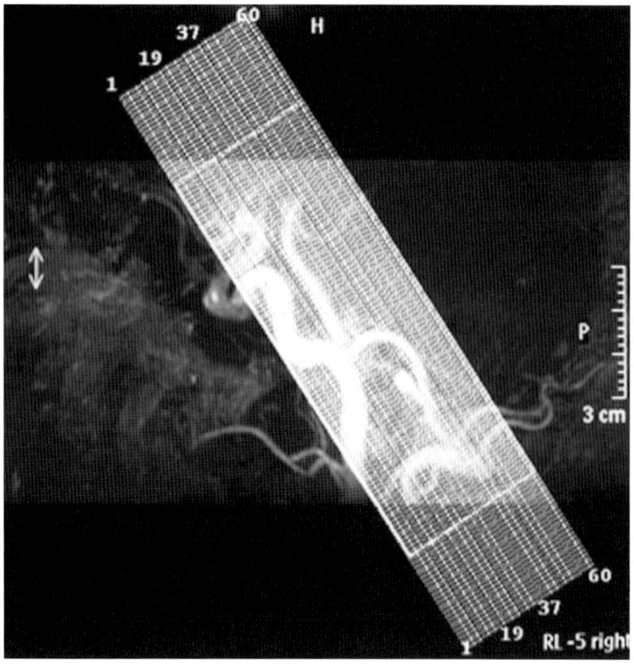

Fig. 1 VISTA was performed as follows: coronal 3D imaging slab centered at the basilar artery was prescribed based on the TOF angiogram

MRI Protocol

MR imaging was performed with a 1.5-T unit (ACHIEVA; Philips Medical Systems, Best, The Netherlands). Cranial MRA was carried out using a 3D TOF technique. Imaging parameters were 24.7/9.6 (TR/TE), 20° flip angle, 150×150-mm field of view, 256×160 matrix, 140 sections with a 0.6-mm effective thickness that resulted in the coverage of a volume of 84 mm in the craniocaudal direction.

BPAS was performed in a 25-mm-thick coronal section parallel to the clivus by using a fast spin-echo sequence. The following imaging parameters were used: 3,000/800 (TR/TE), 150×150-mm field of view, and 256×256 matrix. Acquisition time was 2 min 24 s with our pulse sequence. We added only the gray scale reversal in post-proceedings.

VISTA was performed as follows: the coronal 3D imaging slab centered at the basilar artery was prescribed based on the TOF angiogram (Fig. 1). Refocus control was set up at a 60° angle. ECG triggering was not used. Imaging parameters included: 450/19 (TR/TE), turbo factor 20, 150×150-mm field of view, and a 224×512 matrix. Acquisition time was 5 min 20 s.

Results

On the MRA, pearl-and-string sign was found in two patients, pearl sign in two cases, string sign in four and occlusion in seven. On the BPAS, all but two patients presented with dilatation of the external diameter of the affected artery. By comparing the findings in BPAS with MRA, we could find the discrepancy in 8/15 cases (53%). We could detect intramural hematoma by using VISTA in 10/15 cases (66.7%). Thirteen of fifteen patients received follow-up MRI. Temporal change of arterial shape was confirmed in 7/13 patients (53.8%). On the MRA, occlusive change was detected in one patient, and improvement of the patency in three. On the BPAS, the external dilatation had normalized in four patients. On the VISTA, regression or change in the signal intensity of the intramural hematoma was shown in seven patients (Table 1).

Case 5: A 47-year-old male presented with sudden onset of headache. MRA revealed a string sign, while VISTA showed an intramural hematoma. In this case, we could identify a pseudolumen and narrowed true lumen on VISTA (Fig. 2). He was treated conservatively and underwent follow-up MRI 1 month and 3 months later. VISTA and MRA revealed a normalized artery. On VISTA, the intramural hematoma had regressed. On MRA, the arterial patency had gradually improved. Besides, on BPAS, the external dilatation had normalized (Fig. 3).

Case 12: The 34-year-old male presented with right Wallenberg syndrome. MRA revealed the occlusion of the right VA. VISTA presented an intramural hematoma at the same position. Follow-up MRI was performed 2 and 6 months later. On BPAS, the external dilatation had regressed (Fig. 4).

Case 7: A 46-year-old male presented with headache and left cerebellar infarction. MRA revealed a string sign at the left PICA. BPAS showed dilatation of the external diameter

Table 1 Summary of diagnosis using BPAS and VISTA

Case No.	Age, sex	Presentation	MRA	BPAS	VISTA	Discrepancy MRA and BPAS	Temporal change of arterial shape
1	50F	Headache	Occlusion	Dilatation	–	+	BPAS
2	53F	Headache	Pearl sign	Dilatation	–	–	–
3	52M	Ischemia	Pearl and string	Dilatation	–	–	–
4	64M	Ischemia	Occlusion	Dilatation	Intramural hematoma	+	–
5	47M	Headache	String sign	Dilatation	Intramural hematoma	+	–
6	80F	Headache	Pearl and string	Dilatation	Intramural hematoma	+	MRA, BPAS, VISTA
7	46M	Ischemia	String sign	Dilatation	–	–	–
8	47M	Ischemia	Occlusion	Dilatation	Intramural hematoma	+	VISTA
9	59M	Ischemia	String sign	Dilatation	–	+	–
10	39M	Headache	Occlusion	Dilatation	Intramural hematoma	+	–
11	18M	Ischemia	Occlusion	Normal	Intramural hematoma	–	–
12	34M	Ischemia	Occlusion	Dilatation	Intramural hematoma	+	BPAS, VISTA
13	50M	Ischemia	Oearl sign	Dilatation	Intramural hematoma	–	MRA, VISTA
14	62M	Ischemia	Occlusion	Normal	Intramural hematoma	–	MRA, VISTA
15	38M	Ischemia	String sign	Normal	Intramural hematoma	–	–

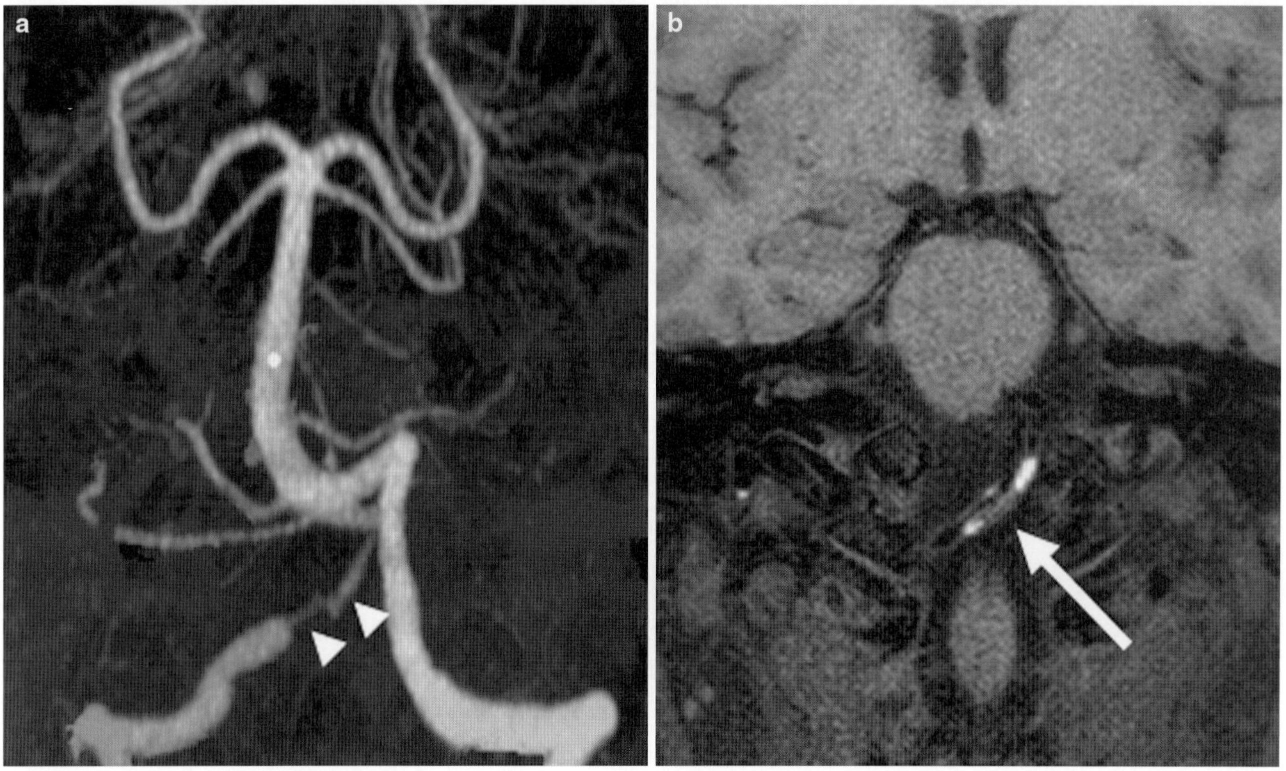

Fig. 2 This 47-year-old male presented with sudden onset of headache. (**a**) MRA revealed a string sign (*arrowhead*), (**b**) VISTA showed an intramural hematoma (*white arrow*). In this case, we could identify the pseudolumen and narrowed true lumen with VISTA

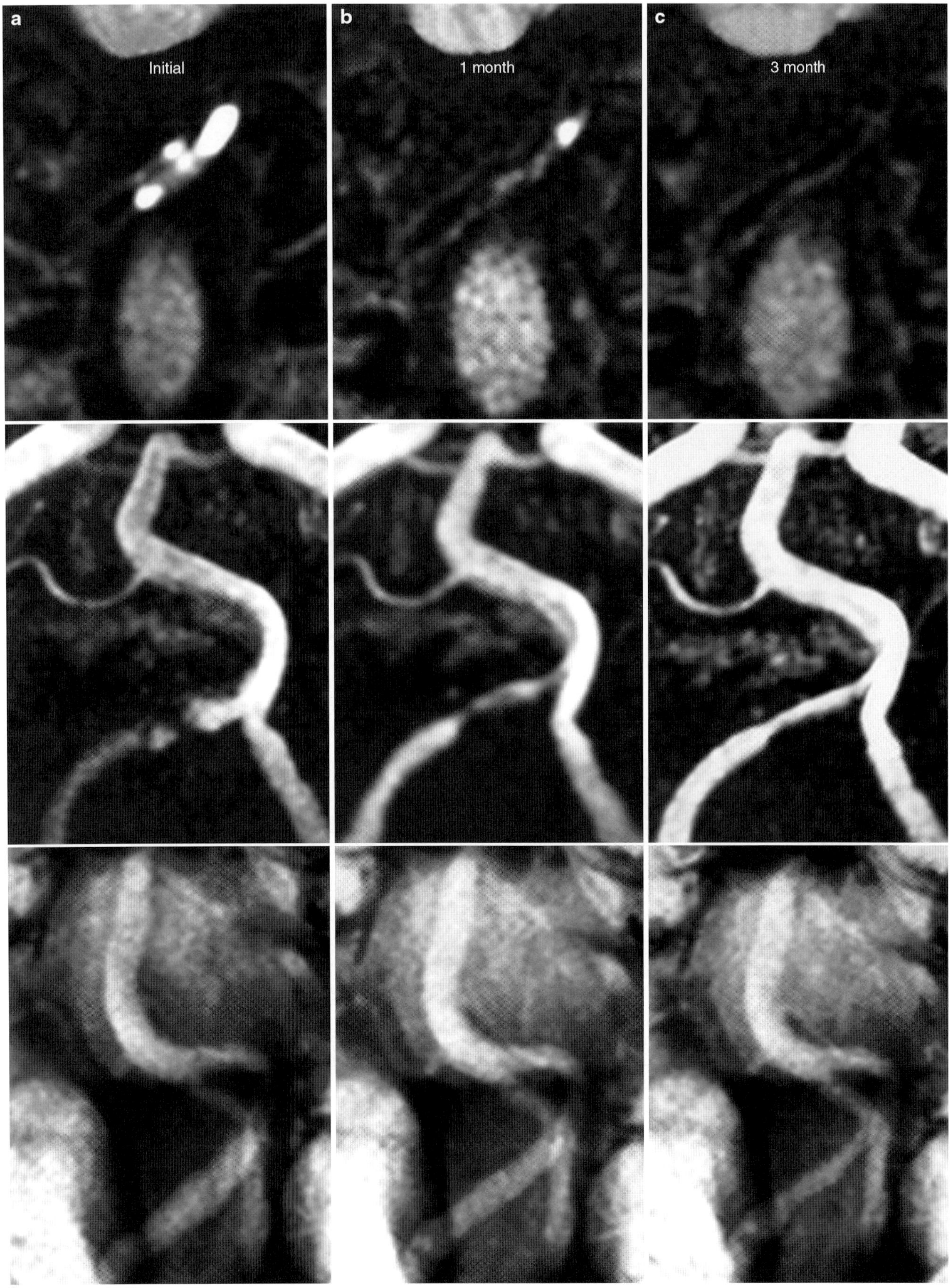

Fig. 3 Initial MRI was performed 2 days after the onset (**a**), follow-up MRI 1 month later (**b**), 3 months later (**c**). VISTA and MRA revealed a normalized artery. On VISTA, the intramural hematoma had regressed. On MRA, the arterial patency had gradually improved. Besides, the external dilatation had normalized on BPAS

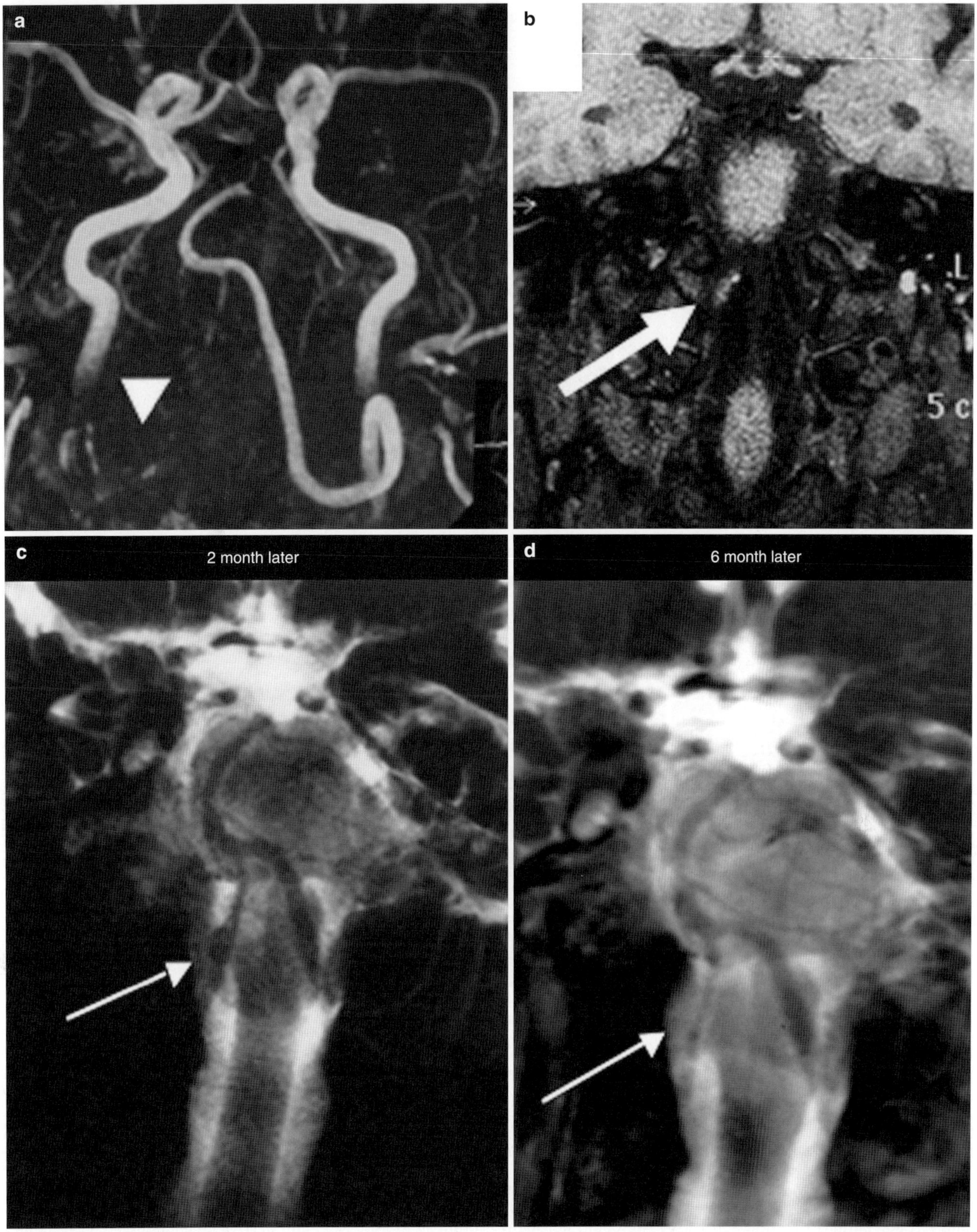

Fig. 4 This 34-year-old male presented with a right Wallenberg syndrome. (**a**) MRA revealed the occlusion of the right VA (*arrowhead*). (**b**) VISTA presented an intramural hematoma at the same position (*large white arrow*). (**c, d**) Follow-up MRI was performed 2 and 6 months later. On BPAS, the external dilatation had regressed (*small white arrow*)

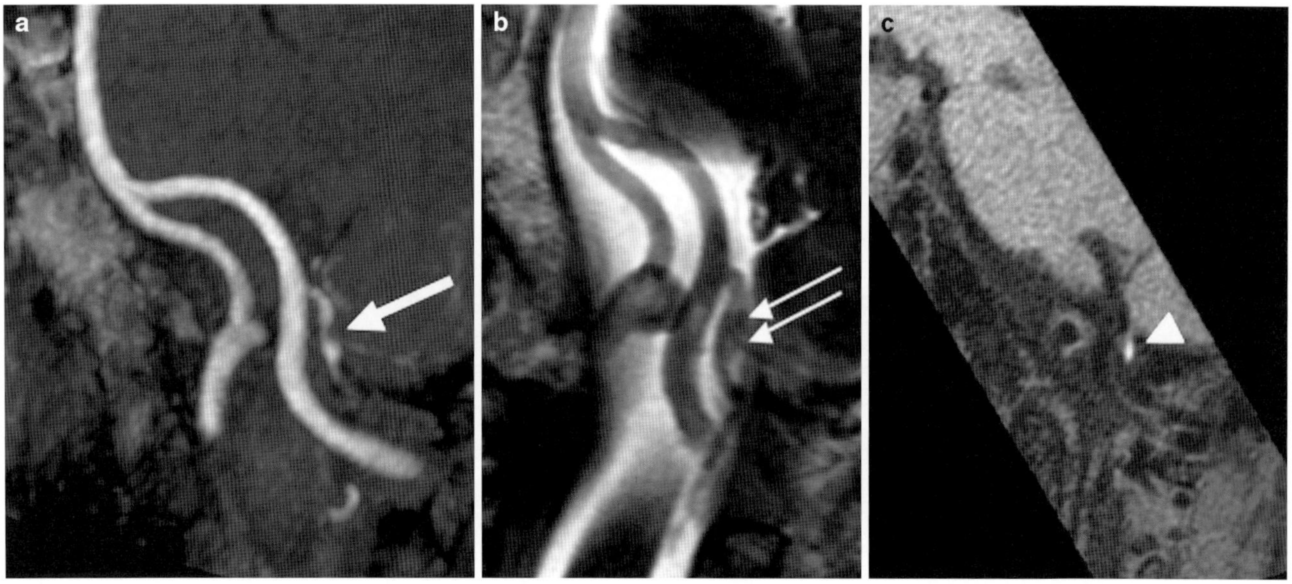

Fig. 5 This 46-year-old male presented with headache and left cerebellar infarction. (**a**) MRA revealed a string sign at the left PICA (*large white arrow*). (**b**) BPAS showed dilatation of external diameter of the vertebral artery (*small white arrow*). (**c**) VISTA indicated an intramural hematoma at the same position (*arrowhead*)

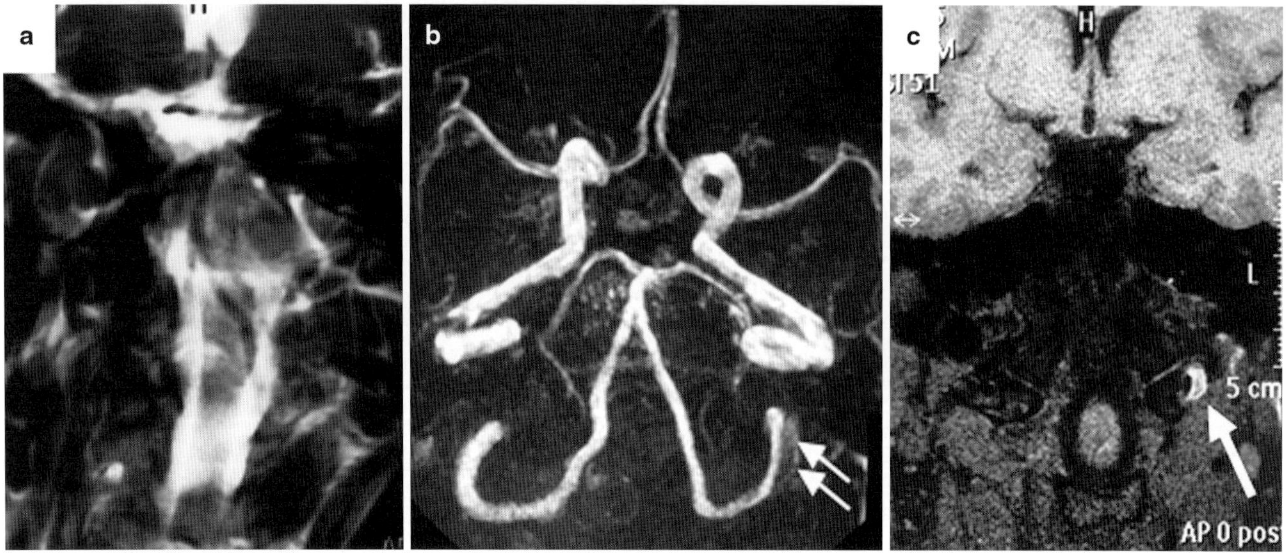

Fig. 6 This 38-year-old male presented with headache and left cerebellar infarction. (**a**) On the BPAS, we could not identify external diameter of vertebral artery, despite our investigation. (**b**) On the MRA, the left vertebral artery was shown in double contrast, which resulted in equivocal findings (*small white arrow*). (**c**) Only VISTA indicated an intramural hematoma at the same position (*large white arrow*)

of the vertebral artery. VISTA indicated an intramural hematoma at the same position (Fig. 5).

Case 15: A 38-year-old male presented with headache and left cerebellar infarction. On BPAS, we could not identify the external diameter of the vertebral artery, although our investigation was possible. On MRA, the left vertebral artery was shown in double contrast, which resulted in equivocal findings. Only VISTA indicated an intramural hematoma at the same position (Fig. 6).

Discussion

Intracranial VA dissections are reported to cause headache, brain stem infarction and SAH with an associated high morbidity and mortality [7, 8]. It has recently drawn attention as a relatively common cause of stroke because of the introduction of MRI as a diagnostic technique [2]. In neuroimaging of dissections, confirming the arterial lumen abnormality was the old standard. Subsequently, intramural hematoma on

MRI has been recognized as the definitive finding [3, 5, 6]. In recent reports, much attention has been paid to the surface appearance of the affected artery.

BPAS-MR imaging can easily show the outer contour of vertebro-basilar arteries clearly. It only requires a 2-cm-thick, heavily T2-weighted coronal imaging, parallel to the clivus, with gray-scale reversal in post-proceedings. By comparing the findings in BPAS with MRA, we can precisely evaluate the condition of the vertebrobasilar artery. Nagahata et al. reported that BPAS was useful to confirm hypoplasia or occluded vertebral arteries, and to reveal the whole appearance of large or partially thrombosed aneurysms of the vertebrobasilar system [4]. It is the same procedure for the dissection. In our study, almost all of the patients presented with dilatation of the external diameter of the affected artery. In addition, a discrepancy between BPAS and MRA and temporal change in their findings were found comparatively frequently, which enabled us to make the diagnosis of dissection. In other words, to perform follow-up MRI as well as MRA with BPAS is recommended for making a diagnosis. With limited use of BPAS, it is difficult to evaluate the outer contour of arteries, which are distant from the median position of clivus. Therefore, it is also hard to evaluate VA dissection distal to the cranio-cervical junction with a single use of BPAS.

VISTA is a sort of black blood imaging method. The feature of the black blood imaging method is to reveal the structure of the arterial wall and lumen clearly. The black blood imaging method has been used in many ways to evaluate carotid plaque [1]. VISTA, which is 3D imaging, enables us to acquire the optimal dimension of the individual vessel. In addition, VISTA does not require the use of the ECG triggering with the refocus control technique. It enables us to shorten the acquisition time and consequently to obtain images with thinner slices as compared with 2D imaging. In our cases, we could identify intramural hematoma by using VISTA in 60%. In contrast to BPAS, it is possible to reveal the structure regardless of laterality.

Conclusion

Dilatation of the external diameter was shown highly frequently in VA dissections. In addition, a discrepancy between BPAS and MRA as well as the intramural hematoma on VISTA was found comparatively frequently. Therefore, performing follow-up MRI is recommended to evaluate the temporal change of the findings for making the diagnosis. BPAS and VISTA are minimally invasive and useful methods for screening tests.

Conflicts of interest statement We declare that we have no conflict of interest.

References

1. Fan Z, Zhang Z, Chung Y et al (2010) Carotid arterial wall MRI at 3T using 3D variable-flip-angle turbo spin-echo (TSE) with flow-sensitive dephasing. J Magn Reson Imaging 31:645–654
2. Leclerc X, Lucas C, Pruvo JP et al (1999) Preliminary experience using contrast-enhanced MR angiography to assess vertebral artery structure for the follow-up of suspected dissection. Am J Neuroradiol 20:1482–1490
3. Lum C, Chakraborty S, Schlossmacher M et al (2009) Vertebral artery dissection with a normal appearing lumen at multisection CT angiography: the importance of identifying wall hematoma. Am J Neuroradiol 30:787–792
4. Nagahata M, Abe Y, Uno S et al (2005) Surface appearance of the vertebrobasilar artery revealed on basiparallel anatomic scanning (BPAS)-MR imaging: Its role for brain MR examination. Am J Neuroradiol 26:2508–2513
5. Ohkuma H, Suzuki S, Kikkawa T et al (2003) Neuroradiologic and clinical features of arterial dissection of the anterior cerebral artery. Am J Neuroradiol 24:691–699
6. Ohkuma H, Suzuki S, Shimamura N et al (2003) Dissecting aneurysms of the middle cerebral artery: neuroradiological and clinical features. Neuroradiology 45:143–148
7. Yamaura A, Watanabe Y, Saeki N (1990) Dissecting aneurysms of the intracranial vertebral artery. J Neurosurg 72:183–188
8. Yoshimoto Y, Wakai S (1997) Unruptured intracranial vertebral artery dissection. Clinical course and serial radiographic imagings. Stroke 28:370–374

Intracranial Stenting in Arterial Occlusive Disease

Bernd Turowski

Abstract The results of endovascular treatment of symptomatic intracranial arteriosclerotic stenosis with stenosis grades exceeding 70% show a mortality rate of 2% and severe morbidity of 8.3%. This justifies treatment being performed by experienced interventionalists only in selected cases, if the prospective outcome of pharmacotherapy alone indicates a higher risk (i.e., symptomatic stenosis, severe perfusion disturbances).

Keywords Intracranial · Stenosis · Stent · Risk analysis

Introduction

The epidemiology of intracranial vascular stenosis is not homogeneously distributed among the world population. Whilst the incidence of intracranial stenosis is 3/100,000 in Europe, it reaches up to 6,000/100,000 in the East Asian population [1].

Risk analysis based on a 50–99% intracranial stenosis reveals a stroke risk of 12–14% within 2 years in symptomatic patients, but it may even exceed 20% per year in individual constellations. Asymptomatic intracranial stenosis seems to bear a very low risk of subsequent stroke. The risk of endovascular treatment is reported to be between 5% and 10% for combined morbidity and mortality [2].

B. Turowski
Department of Neurosurgery, Heinrich Heine University, Moorenstraße 5, 40225 Düsseldorf, Germany
e-mail: bernd.turowski@uni-duesseldorf.de

Materials and Methods

In our institution, we consider endovascular treatment of intracranial stenosis if there are recurrent clinical symptoms despite best medical treatment related to the stenosis, and if the degree of stenosis exceeds 70%. Additionally, in individual cases, we consider revascularization if there are severe disturbances of perfusion and if no vascular reserve in the acetazolamide challenge is present. In addition, a passage of stenosis with a microguidewire must technically be possible.

Based on conventional angiography, the degree, length and anatomy of the stenosis is defined. In all cases, stent-assisted angioplasty is performed. If balloon-mounted stents are used, they are principally undersized by around 10% [3]. A stable coaxial access (long sheath + guiding catheter) is essential for complete control during the intervention.

Data of 48 patients were collected from four hospitals collaborating in this study. Predilatation was used in 38/48 stenoses. After endovascular treatment, supervision of the patient with strict control of the systolic blood pressure is necessary in all cases. Location of stenosis was:

ACI (intracranial): 8 patients
MCA: 8 patients
VA: 17 patients
BA: 15 patients

Results

The mean value of the extent of stenosis was reduced from 89% (range 70–99%) to 24.5% after endovascular treatment. Thirty-day mortality was 1/48 (2%) because of a reperfusion hemorrhage. Severe morbidity occurred in 4/48 (8.3%) correlated to: one reperfusion hemorrhage, one mesencephalic infarction, one MCA infarction, and one ACP infarction after lysis of basilar thrombosis. Mild morbidity was found in 2/48 (4.2%), corresponding to one fluctuating dysarthria and one mild aggravation of dysarthria.

T. Tsukahara et al. (eds.), *Trends in Neurovascular Surgery*, Acta Neurochirurgica Supplementum, Vol. 112,
DOI: 10.1007/978-3-7091-0661-7_12, © Springer-Verlag/Wien 2011

Discussion

In selected cases with strong indications, risk analysis shows a benefit for stent-assisted intracranial angioplasty. Especially in the collective of patients with severe vasculopathia, intracranial stent-assisted angioplasty may be a technical challenge requiring experience and suitable material. It is an effective treatment that will become safer with technical progress. Postinterventional blood pressure management is essential to avoid reperfusion hemorrhages.

Conflict of interest statement We declare that we have no conflict of interest.

References

1. Fareed M, Suri S, Claiborne Johnston (2009) Epidemiology of intracranial stenosis. J Neuroimaging 19(S1):11–16
2. Lutsep HL, Barnwell SL, Mawad M, SSYLVIA Study investigators (2004) Stenting of symptomatic sclerotic lesions in the vertebral or intracranial arteries (SSYLVIA). Stroke 35(6):1388–1392
3. Rochemont RduM, Turowski B, Buchkremer M, Sitzer M, Zanella FE, Berkefeld J (2004) Recurrent symptomatic high-grade intracranial stenoses: safety and efficacy of undersized stents – initial experience. Radiology 231(1):45–49

Treatment of Aneurysms and Subarachnoid Hemorrhage

A View on the Current and Future Therapy of Brain Aneurysms

Hans-Jakob Steiger

Abstract While in clinical practice the use of endovascular and microsurgical methods retained relative levels by 2010, since 2008 the research activity has lagged behind that in other medical disciplines. Particularly research on neuroprotection, such as hypothermia and pharmacological measures, has lost impetus, and clinical applications of specific neuroprotective interventions have been largely abandoned. The last substantial advancement for aneurysm surgery was the introduction of intraoperative indocyanine green (ICG) angiography. The technical evolution of endovascular therapy has been somewhat more active than that of microsurgery. It is our conviction that microsurgical methods need to develop a focus particularly on minimal invasiveness and also cosmetic aspects. Teaching remains an important consideration. It appears that an explicit framework is necessary in order to communicate the specific do's, don'ts and hows of aneurysm surgery, i.e., a set of rules addressing general perioperative management, principles of exposure and dissection of the typical configurations, clipping technique and the specific issues concerning very small and very large aneurysms. Quality management has become an unconditional requirement also in neurovascular surgery. At our department we have established a system of identification of complications and monthly case analysis. Despite these efforts combined management morbidity and mortality for ruptured and unruptured aneurysms remains around 10%, which appears to be the achievable degree of safety in unselected patients with the current technology.

H.-J. Steiger
Department of Neurosurgery, Heinrich Heine University, Moorenstraße 5, 40225 Düsseldorf, Germany
e-mail: steiger@uni-duesseldorf.de

Keywords Brain aneurysm · Subarachnoid hemorrhage · Neurovascular research · Teaching · Quality management

Framework for Aneurysm Surgery 2010

While during the last decade knowledge and proficiency with regard to the microsurgical treatment of posterior circulation aneurysms has been lost without discussion and beyond reasonable doubt, the issue of giant aneurysms is still open to some degree, partially because the topic is less concise than the basilar bifurcation aneurysm, and multiple arguments play a role during decision making with regard to the best way of managing a ruptured or unruptured giant aneurysm.

The evolution of endovascular stents has certainly opened new and less invasive ways to manage even large broad-based and fusiform aneurysms while preserving parent arteries. Although bypass surgery for giant and fusiform aneurysms has always been practiced only at a few centers, this kind of surgery appears to be rarely indicated nowadays.

With regard to small- and medium-sized saccular aneurysms, endovascular and microsurgical treatments are balanced, and both modalities are used in synergy if the whole picture needs to be considered. No neurosurgeon in 2010 would want to be without endovascular therapy. Without doubt, there are still competing aspects in the interaction between neurosurgery and endovascular therapy, but a number of secondary analyses of the ISAT and ISUIA data have provided peace of mind for both groups as they proposed balanced subgroups of patients who would benefit from endovascular therapy or microsurgery, respectively. For example, the subanalysis of the ISAT data by Mitchell and co-workers suggested that young and elderly patients with ruptured aneurysms should be treated microsurgically, while the middle-aged group would benefit from endovascular treatment [2].

DOI: 10.1007/978-3-7091-0661-7_13,

Current Scientific Position on SAH and Aneurysm Research

After having clarified the synergies between the treatment modalities, the more important topic is the position of SAH and brain aneurysms in research. In order to get a grasp on the actual position of these themes in medical research, we conducted a PubMed search with the keywords "subarachnoid hemorrhage" and "brain aneurysm," and compared the development of the respective proportion of all PubMed entries over the last decade (Fig. 1). While the total number of PubMed entries increased linearly at a rate of some 5% per year, the yearly output with the keyword "subarachnoid hemorrhage" increased at approximately the same rate until 2008, but has been stagnating since then. With regard to publications with the keyword "brain aneurysm," a substantial decline at a rate of 10% per year has been noticed since 2008. From this analysis we must conclude that medical progress is more active in other fields and that, on the whole, progress has stagnated in the field of aneurysm and SAH research.

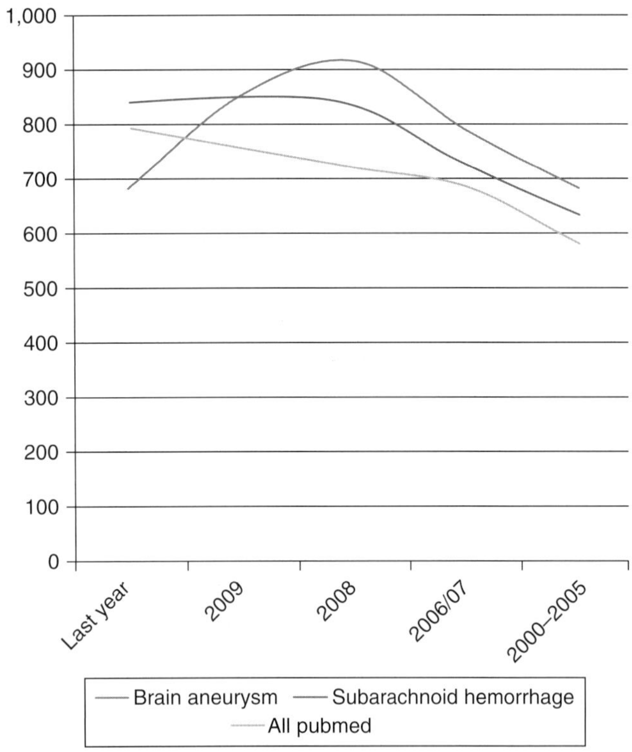

Fig. 1 Current scientific position of SAH and aneurysm research. Development of PubMed entries over the last decade with the key words "subarachnoid hemorrhage" and "brain aneurysm" respectively, in comparison with the overall PubMed evolution

Uncertainties and Trends Regarding Treatment of Brain Aneurysms in 2010

To be more specific, what are the central considerations with regard to aneurysm and SAH management in 2010?

- Endovascular therapy is accepted as the first choice after SAH.
- Vasospasm is still an issue, although undoubtedly progress has been made.
- Genetic factors are still incompletely understood.
- Treatment indications for unruptured aneurysms need further clarification.

Traditionally the following statements have been expressed with regard to the impact of the advent of endovascular therapy on neurosurgical management:

- More difficult aneurysms are referred for surgery.
- Surgery can avoid risky maneuvers.

While these positions cannot be considered wrong in principle, they are certainly not absolute. Essentially, these positions are contradictory, but in real life they lead to the necessary balance.

The Necessity of Continuing Technical Evolution in Aneurysm Microsurgery

There is no doubt that with regard to the small aneurysms, there is continuing competition between the methods. Nonetheless, one need not be clairvoyant to see that microsurgical management will disappear if no major progress is made in microsurgical technology. While the long-term results expressed as rerupture rates have hardly varied, the invasiveness of the treatment modality and cosmetic aspects have gained in importance. Therefore, at our center we have introduced minimally invasive custom-tailored approaches for the specific aneurysms, and we have completely abandoned the universal grand pterional craniotomy. Of course, safety is the most important aspect in aneurysm surgery. However, the size of the craniotomy does not automatically also indicate its safety, and vice versa. In retrospect, the development of the small orbito-craniotomy for the anterior communicating artery complex and the small sylvian craniotomy for the middle cerebral artery must be considered successful modifications [6]. The orbitocraniotomy allows for a more ventral access to the anterior communicating artery with the potential to avoid damage to the frontal lobe and particularly the gyrus rectus. With the small sylvian approach to the middle cerebral artery bifurcation, the sylvian fissure is split from peripheral to central, and proximal control of M1 is usually gained between the M2 trunks. This approach largely avoids necessary retraction of the frontal lobe in order to first control the proximal M1.

While these two developments have proved to be beneficial and practical, it is not enough. At our center, a number of other concepts have been followed over the years. Many have proved not to be feasible or to provide no benefit. For example, for some time we evaluated the use of neuronavigation for aneurysm surgery, but had to accept that with the current degree of precision, navigation does not help.

Technological research and development in endovascular therapy have been more active. New coils and stents are still being developed. Microsurgery can benefit from some of the neuroradiological developments. The better quality angiography and CT angiography help to obtain a clear image of the vascular anatomy prior to surgery. We should also routinely make use of the 3D tools in order to plan our neurosurgical procedures exactly.

Intraoperative imaging with indocyanine green (ICG) is one recent technological improvement in vascular microneurosurgery. ICG angiography has become accepted as a useful tool for aneurysms, AVM and bypass. Here the development is still in progress. Current prototypes allow for dynamic ICG imaging and calculation of transit curves, thus allowing for regional cerebral blood flow analysis under the surgical microscope (Fig. 2).

What happened to intraoperative neuroprotection? Hypothermia, barbiturates and Suzuki's cocktail have become unpopular, at least in Europe, because these methods require dedicated neuroanesthetists. With the development toward high put-through surgery in the last decade, the processes had to be rationalized. Since we never had any evidence for

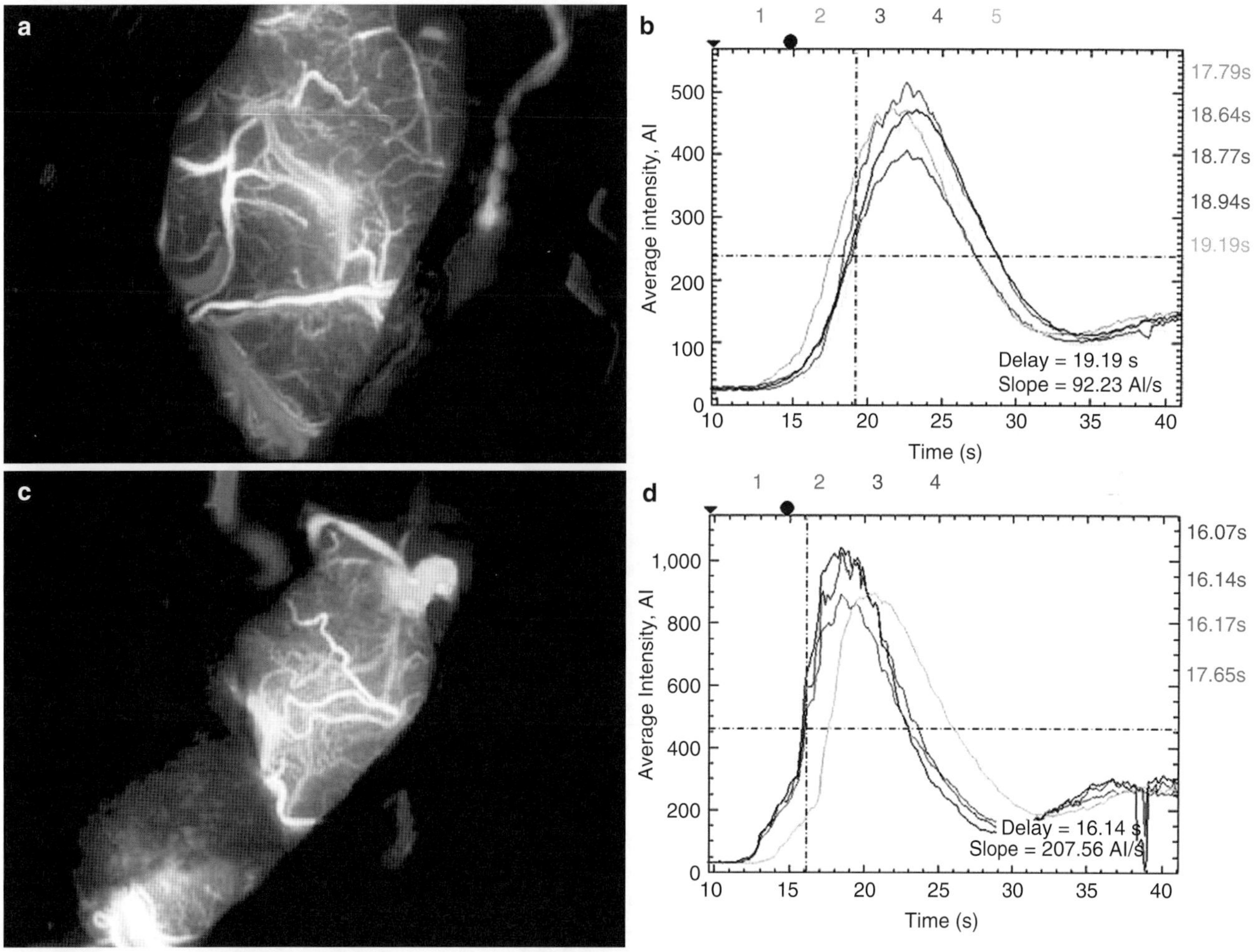

Fig. 2 Intraoperative dynamic ICG angiography. Quantitative tracking of the ICG bolus allows calculating regional perfusion indices. (**a**) Cortical ICG angiography in a case of internal carotid artery occlusion. (**b**) Dynamic ICG passage through different regions of interest (ROIs). (**c**) Cortical ICG angiography after EC-IC bypass. (**d**) Graph of the ICG passage through the different ROIs shows shortening of the transit times, a shift to the left

the benefit of intraoperative neuroprotective anesthesia, such as hypothermia, magnesium, barbiturates, etc. [4], it was easy to abandon these adjuvant measures. Independent of the use of neuroprotective measures, the known ischemic tolerances of the concerned arterial territories must be kept in mind when using temporary clips.

Intraoperative neurophysiologic monitoring (IOM) for aneurysm surgery never gained widespread acceptance, although the evidence level is not worse than that of other branches of neurosurgery where IOM is firmly established [3]. The fact that aneurysm surgery is usually not elective likely plays the most important role. This situation is comparable to the lack of acceptance of neuronavigation for insertion of ventricular drains and shunts.

Teaching Issues

Teaching aneurysm surgery remains an important aspect. The cornerstones of efficient teaching remain the same:

- Training environment
- Teacher dedication
- Structured syllabus

Nonetheless, some differences to former generations have become apparent in today's teaching environment. While some young colleagues appear to learn the essentials very quickly, others repeatedly make mistakes that teachers have not considered. Therefore, an explicit framework appears to be necessary in order to communicate the specific do's, don'ts and hows. From one point of view, the ideal candidates for successful and rapid training in aneurysm surgery are already experienced microsurgeons who want to expand their expertise to aneurysm surgery. In practice, this condition is uncommon and also has disadvantages. The main problem is that these colleagues rarely have a specific scientific interest in vascular neurosurgery and therefore also face natural limits for their surgical format. The prototype of the experienced microneurosurgeon is, however, interesting from the didactic point of view, because the essentials of aneurysm surgery can be communicated to this group with a clear set of rules addressing general perioperative management, principles of exposure and dissection of the typical configurations, clipping technique and the specific issues concerning very small and very large aneurysms.

More commonly, the trainee is a senior resident or junior staff member who still requires some training in microsurgical techniques. Nonetheless, it is our conviction that the ability to express the essentials of aneurysm surgery in words is essential for successful training [5]. For example, the typology of aneurysm configurations used at Heinrich Heine University (HHU) will be mentioned. For the typical aneurysm locations, we have defined the four prevailing projections, because these projections govern the approach and dissection (Fig. 3). Based on the projection, the approach to

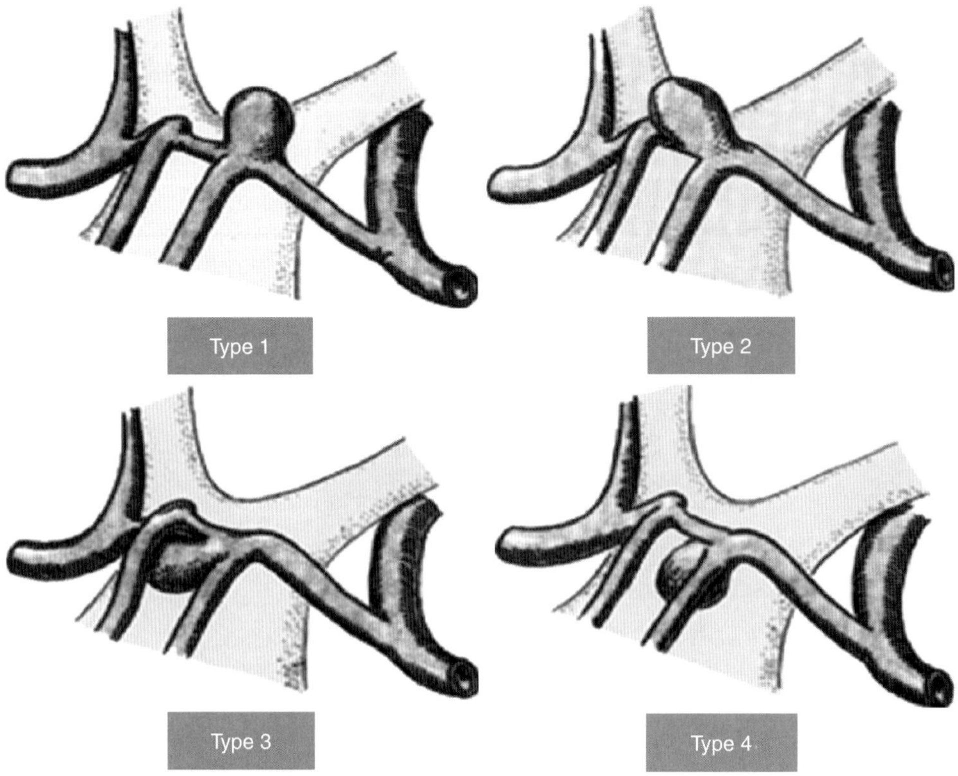

Fig. 3 Classification of anterior communicating artery aneurysms used at our department for teaching purposes. It is our conviction that the specifics of aneurysm surgery need to be explained explicitly, which requires a concise framework of aneurysm types

the aneurysm is specified during the preoperative briefing. Depending on the degree of competency, the senior neurosurgeon can then join the operation during the dissection phase.

Quality Management

At HHU we have developed a reasonably reliable process to encode and retrieve management complications [7]. Encoding is based on an outcome classification that is transcribed in plain language also in the discharge summary. Therefore, correct encoding is verified by the patients and relatives as well as all the physicians involved in the care of the patients. Cross-checks indicate that for elective cases complications are identified with a sensitivity of more than 90%. However, reliable management related morbidity and mortality (M&M) data is currently only available for elective neurovascular cases (unruptured aneurysm, dural arteriovenous fistula, AVM, elective bypass). For SAH and ruptured AVM management, morbidity is obscured by the impact of the initial hemorrhage [1].

Complications are discussed at HHU Department of Neurosurgery in a monthly Morbidity & Mortality (M&M) teaching conference. Over the last years the rate of complications of aneurysm and SAH management has remained stable. The 2009 figures for registered morbidity and mortality are given in Fig. 4. The rates fluctuate to some degree, but there is no evident trend of continuing improvement. The actual numbers therefore appear to represent a steady state reflecting the current limits of medicine. This statement is not intended to question the importance of the M&M conferences. The M&M conference is an excellent problem-oriented teaching session that is essential for training residents and fellows.

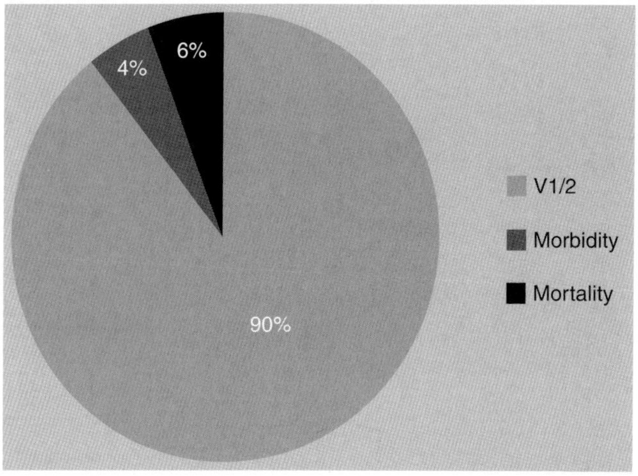

Fig. 4 Morbidity and mortality rates of patients with clipped ruptured and unruptured aneurysms in 2009 at HHU. V1 signifies a positive hospital course with resolution of symptoms and deficits. V2 specifies a course as expected with stable symptoms and deficits. Mortality includes all lethal cases and also patients dying as a consequence of a poor grade SAH. Morbidity includes all management-related negative side effects of treatment

Conclusions

Scientific activity concerning SAH falls slightly short of general medical scientific progress. Technical aspects of aneurysm surgery have advanced only little in the last years. Surgical and endovascular indications depend on local preconditions. Attention to cosmetic and minimally invasive aspects is crucial for the future of the microsurgical method. An explicit framework for the essentials of aneurysm surgery appears to be important for efficient training. Current technology does not seem to be able to reduce the actual M&M rates significantly further in unselected aneurysm patients.

Conflict of interest statement We declare that we have no conflict of interest.

References

1. Lawton MT, Du R, Tran MN, Achrol AS, McCulloch CE, Johnston SC, Quinnine NJ, Young WL (2005) Effect of presenting hemorrhage on outcome after microsurgical resection of brain arteriovenous malformations. Neurosurgery 56:485–493
2. Mitchell P, Kerr R, Mendelow AD, Molyneux A (2008) Could late rebleeding overturn the superiority of cranial aneurysm coil embolization over clip ligation seen in the International Subarachnoid Aneurysm Trial? J Neurosurg 108:437–442
3. Neuloh G, Schramm J (2004) Monitoring of motor evoked potentials compared with somatosensory evoked potentials and microvascular Doppler ultrasonography in cerebral aneurysm surgery. J Neurosurg 100:389–399
4. Schmid-Elsaesser R, Kunz M, Zausinger S, Prueckner S, Briegel J, Steiger HJ (2006) Intravenous magnesium versus nimodipine in the treatment of patients with aneurysmal subarachnoid hemorrhage: a randomized study. Neurosurgery 58:1054–1065
5. Sennet R (2008) The craftsman. Part II craft, expressive instructions. Yale University Press, New Haven
6. Steiger HJ, Schmid-Elsaesser R, Stummer W, Uhl E (2001) Transorbital keyhole approach to anterior communicating artery aneurysms. Neurosurgery 48(2):347–351
7. Steiger HJ, Stummer W, Hänggi D (2010) Can systematic analysis of morbidity and mortality reduce surgical complication rates in neurosurgery. Acta Neurochir 152:2013–2019

Surgical Treatment for Aneurysms in the Cavernous – Petrous Portion of the Internal Carotid Artery

Hiroshi Abe, Koichiro Takemoto, Toshio Higashi, and Tooru Inoue

Abstract *Background*: As direct surgery to treat aneurysms in the cavernous-petrous portion of the ICA is difficult, proximal ligation of the ICA with or without bypass surgery is still the conventional treatment. Some patients have an ECA-ICA collateral pathway distal to the ligation site. This is related to the recanalization of the aneurysm. We describe the treatment strategy of these aneurysms and the surgical pitfalls of the treatment.

Methods: We analyzed 30 cases of symptomatic aneurysms in the cavernous-petrous portion of the ICA. In all cases, proximal ligation of the ICA was performed with bypass surgery followed by BTO.

Results: In 21 patients who could tolerate BTO, we performed a low-flow bypass. In nine patients who could not tolerate BTO, we performed a high-flow bypass. In four patients with ECA-ICA collateral pathways distal to the ligation site, we performed endovascular parent artery occlusion using detachable coils. In four patients without endovascular parent artery occlusion, we experienced recanalization of the aneurysm.

Conclusion: Based on our experience and in view of the late recanalization of aneurysms that have an ECA-ICA collateral pathway, we recommend that intraoperative angiography should be performed to detect the ECA-ICA collateral pathway in proximal ligation of the ICA.

Keywords Internal carotid artery aneurysm · Cavernous sinus · Bypass surgery · Collateral pathway

H. Abe (✉), K. Takemoto, T. Higashi, and T. Inoue
Department of Neurosurgery, Fukuoka University,
7-45-1 Nanakuma, Jonan-ku, Fukuoka 814-0180, Japan
e-mail: hiroshiabe@aol.com

Introduction

As direct surgery to treat large and giant aneurysms in the cavernous-petrous portion of the internal carotid artery (ICA) is difficult, proximal ligation of the ICA with or without bypass surgery is still the conventional treatment. Concurrent with the advances in endovascular techniques, many diagnostic tests have been developed to evaluate the risk of ischemic infarction from carotid occlusion before permanent ICA sacrifice. The most widely accepted tool is clinical balloon test occlusion (BTO) [3, 7, 9].

We did not perform proximal ligation without bypass because BTO has the same false-negative results. We use clinical BTO to choose between the low-flow and high-flow bypass. After proximal ligation of the ICA, in some patients the external carotid artery (ECA)-ICA collateral pathway is distal to the ligation site [6]. This is related to the recanalization of the ICA or aneurysm. We describe the treatment strategy of these aneurysms and the surgical pitfalls of the treatment.

Materials and Methods

From 1988 – 2010, a total of 30 aneurysms in the cavernous-petrous portion of the ICA were treated at our department. Patients included 7 males and 22 females ranging in age from 28 to 78 years (mean, 61.7 years). One patient had bilateral ICA aneurysms. Three lesions were located in the petrous ICA, and 27 in the cavernous ICA. All patients had some symptoms, such as diplopia, orbital pain and nasal bleeding.

All patients underwent and passed a 15-min clinical BTO, including a cerebral blood flow (CBF) study. In patients who tolerated BTO, a superficial temporal artery (STA)-middle cerebral artery (MCA) bypass was performed followed by ICA ligation. In patients who could not tolerate BTO, a radial

DOI: 10.1007/978-3-7091-0661-7_14, © Springer-Verlag/Wien 2011

artery (RA)-middle cerebral artery second portion (M2) bypass was performed followed by ICA ligation. After the above surgical procedure, intra- or postoperative DSA was performed. When the DSA demonstrated no filling of the ICA, we chose careful observation. When the DSA demonstrated filling of the ICA after ligation, we considered that there was an ECA-ICA collateral pathway. In patients who had an ECA-ICA collateral pathway, direct puncture of the ICA distal to the ligation site and parent artery occlusion (PAO) using detachable coils were performed, usually in one stage (Fig. 1).

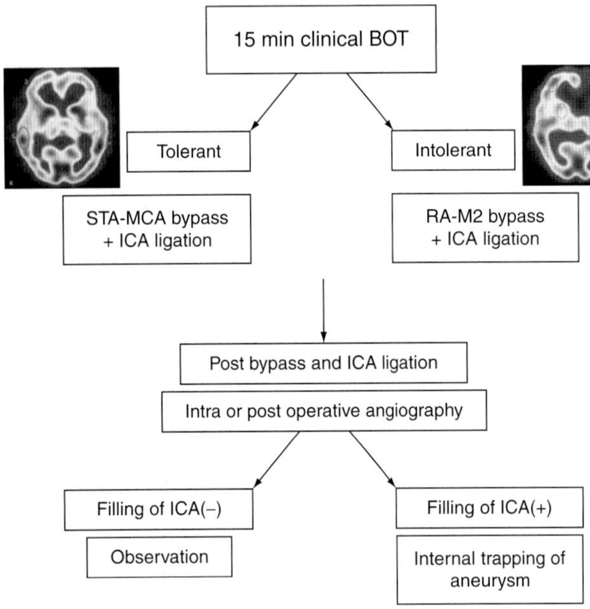

Fig. 1 Management algorithm for large or giant cavernous-petrous aneurysms in the internal carotid artery

Representative Cases

Case 1

A 58-year-old female presented with right oculomotor and abducens palsy. Magnetic resonance imaging disclosed a mass lesion in the right cavernous sinus (Fig. 2). Right carotid angiography revealed a giant cavernous sinus aneurysm. This patient could tolerate BOT. STA-MCA bypass was performed followed by ICA ligation. Intraoperative DSA showed filling of the petrous ICA. Endovascular PAO was performed immediately during the surgical procedure. Postoperative DSA showed no filling of the petrous ICA.

Case 2

A 76-year-old female presented with right oculomotor palsy. Angiography showed a giant right intracavernous ICA aneurysm (Fig. 3). This patient could not tolerate BOT. An RA-M2 bypass was performed followed by ICA ligation. Intraoperative DSA showed no filling of the ICA. However, 4 days after the operation, she presented with hemiparesis and consciousness disturbance. DSA showed good patency of the RA-M2 bypass; antegrade recanalization of the ICA via an ECA was revealed.

Case 3

A 58-year-old female presented with left oculomotor and abducens palsy and orbital pain. 3D-CTA showed a giant

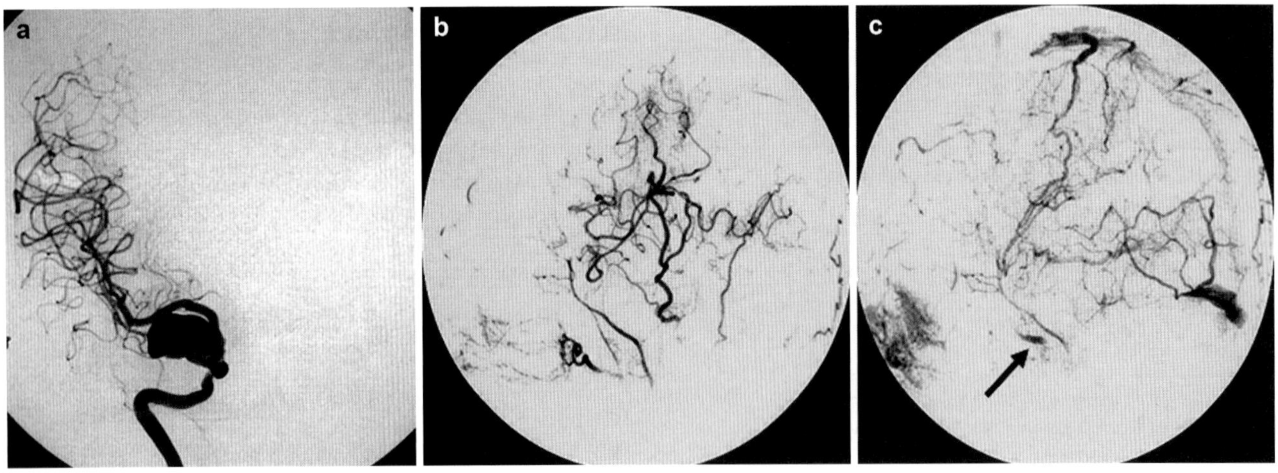

Fig. 2 Case 1. (**a**) Preoperative right carotid angiogram demonstrating a giant cavernous sinus aneurysm. (**b**) Early phase of intraoperative right carotid angiogram showing good patency of the low-flow bypass. (**c**) Late phase of intraoperative right carotid angiogram showing filling of the petrous ICA (*black arrow*). (**d**) Endovascular parent artery occlusion was performed immediately during the surgical procedure (*white arrow*). (**e**) Postoperative right carotid angiogram showing no filling of the petrous ICA

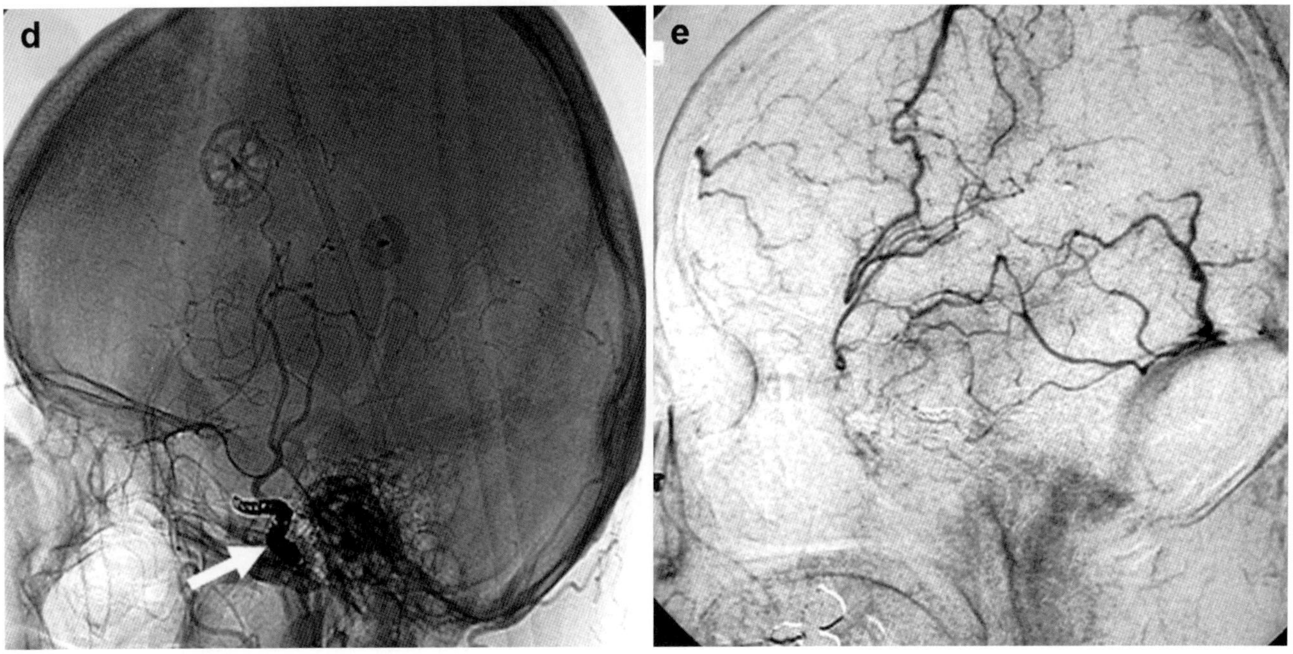

Fig. 2 (continued)

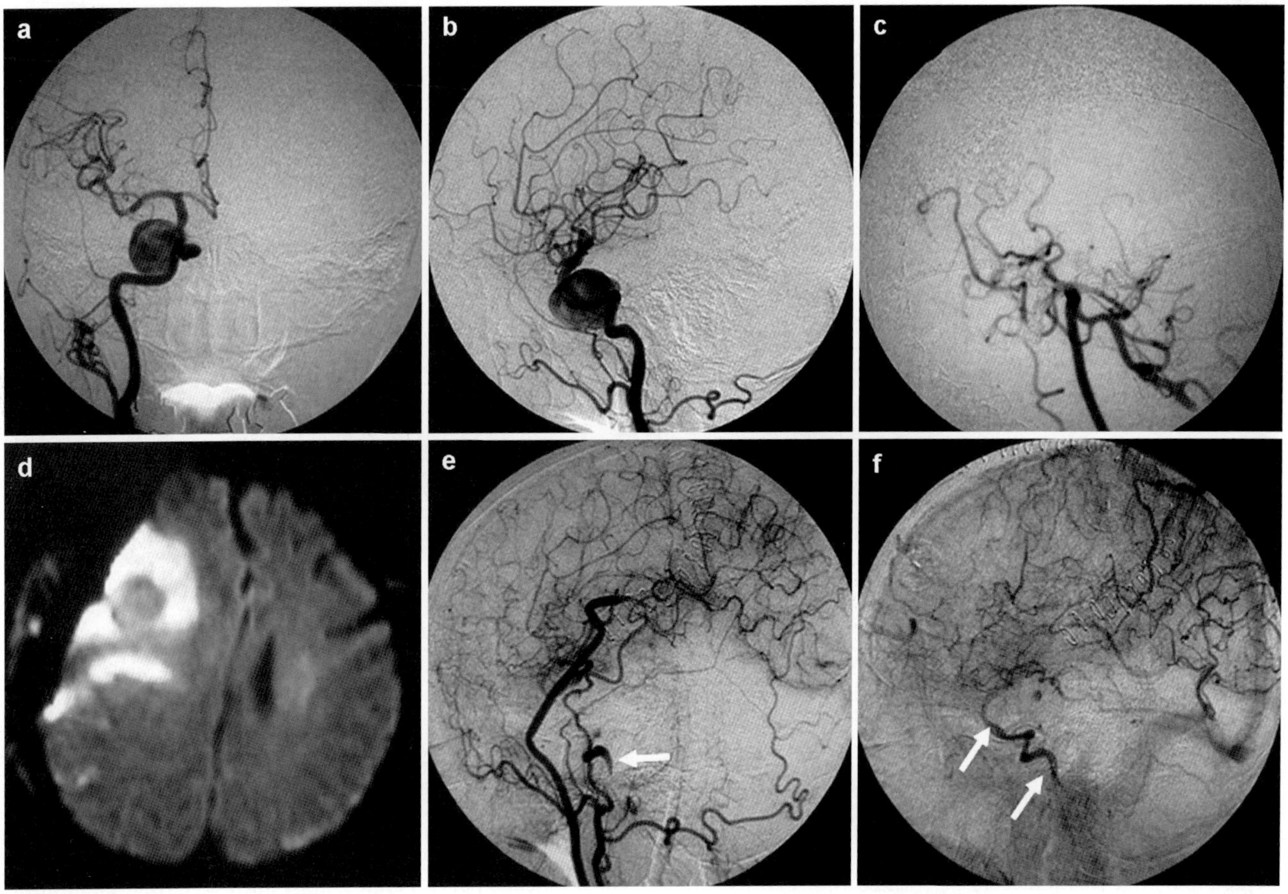

Fig. 3 Case 2. (**a**, **b**) Preoperative right carotid angiogram demonstrating an intracavernous aneurysm. (**c**) Postoperative right carotid angiogram showing good patency of the high-flow bypass and no filling of the ICA. (**d**) Diffusion-weighted image 4 days after the operation showing high signal intensity in the territory of the middle cerebral artery. (**e**) Early phase of postoperative right carotid angiogram showing good patency of RA-M2 bypass. (**f**) Late phase of postoperative right carotid angiogram showing antegrade recanalization of the ICA (*white arrow*)

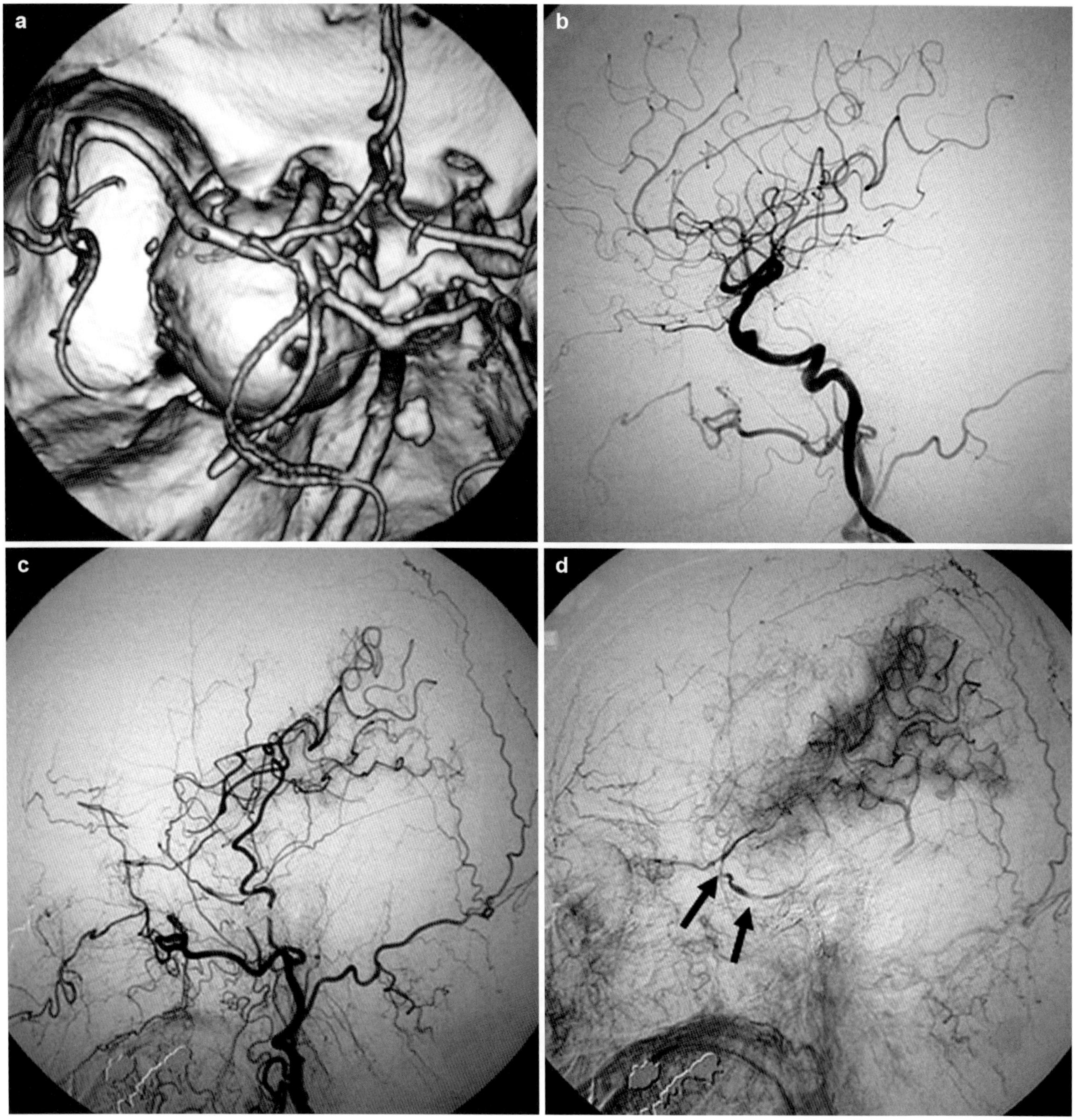

Fig. 4 Case 3. (**a**) Preoperative 3D-CT angiogram showing a giant aneurysm in the left cavernous sinus. (**b**) Preoperative left carotid angiogram demonstrating a partially thrombosed giant cavernous sinus aneurysm. (**c**, **d**) Postoperative left carotid angiogram showing filling of the ICA in a position distal to the coil packing (*black arrow*)

aneurysm in the left cavernous sinus (Fig. 4). Left carotid angiography revealed a partially thrombosed giant cavernous sinus aneurysm. This patient tolerated BOT. STA-MCA bypass and ICA ligation were performed followed by endovascular PAO. Intraoperative DSA showed no filling of the ICA. However, postoperative DSA showed filling of the ICA in a position distal to the coil packing. We chose careful observation because recanalization showed slow retrograde flow.

Case 4

A 56-year-old female presented with right oculomotor and abducens palsy. Angiography showed a right giant intracavernous ICA aneurysm (Fig. 5). This patient did not tolerate BOT. High-flow bypass was performed followed by ICA ligation. Postoperative angiography showed no filling of the aneurysm. One month later, the patient's symptoms

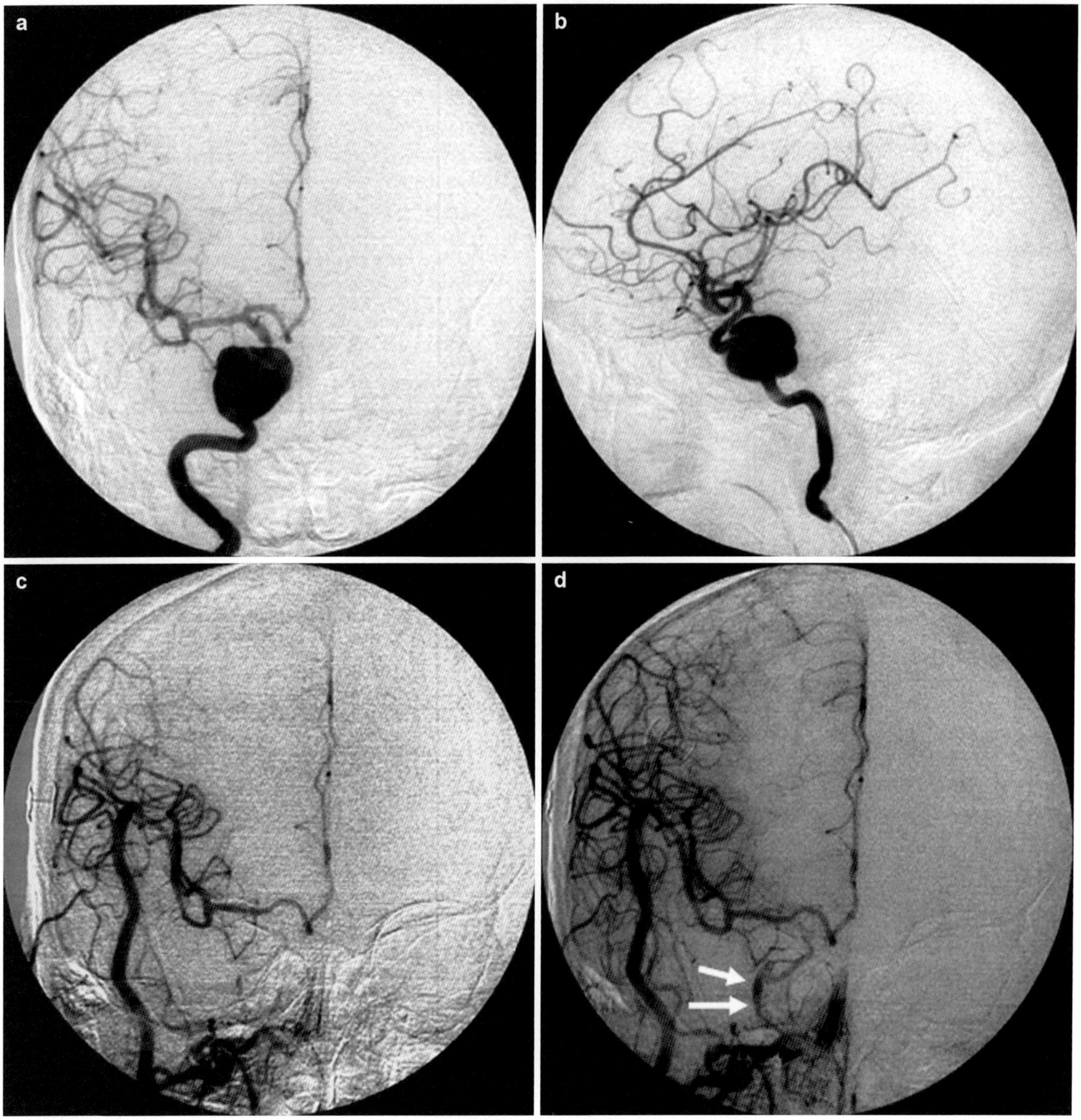

Fig. 5 Case 4. (**a**, **b**) Preoperative right carotid angiogram demonstrating a giant intracavernous aneurysm. (**c**) Postoperative right carotid angiogram showing no filling of the aneurysm. (**d**) Postoperative right carotid angiogram 1 month after the operation demonstrating retrograde recanalization of the ICA due to backflow of the RA graft

had become exacerbated, and angiography demonstrated recanalization of the ICA due to backflow of the RA graft. Endovascular PAO was performed via RA.

Results

In 21 patients who tolerated BTO, we performed a low-flow bypass. In nine patients who could not tolerate BTO, we performed a high-flow bypass with RA graft. In 24 patients we performed intraoperative angiography, and in 4 patients who had an ECA-ICA collateral pathway distal to the ligation site, we performed endovascular parent artery occlusion using detachable coils. The postoperative angiogram showed the arterial bypass to be widely patent in all cases. In 26 patients the aneurysms thrombosed and decreased in size. In four patients without endovascular parent artery occlusion, we experienced recanalization of the aneurysm. The causes of ICA recanalization were backflow of the RA-M2 bypass in two patients, slack at the ligation site in one patient and the ECA-ICA collateral pathway in five patients. Treatments for recanalization of the ICA were surgical trapping of the ICA in one patient, endovascular PAO in six and observation in one. Ischemic complications were found to be due to recanalization of the ICA in two patients. These ischemic complications may have been caused by artery-to-artery embolism. None of the patients experienced infarction with the endovascular procedure.

The recurrent aneurysm and the recanalized internal carotid artery were treated by endovascular procedures. Following surgical carotid artery exposure, direct puncture of the internal carotid artery distal to the site of ligation was achieved. The recanalized internal carotid artery and aneurysm were occluded using detachable coils without anticoagulation therapy. We did not experience complications due to endovascular treatment during the surgical procedure.

Discussion

Historically, direct clipping of cavernous ICA aneurysms has been performed [2]. Although direct clipping can preserve the antegrade blood flow of the ICA, there are many risks of cranial nerve and brain injury. ICA proximal ligations without bypass for ICA aneurysms have been reported. The morbidity and mortality rate of patients whose intracranial ICA aneurysms were treated by ICA ligation was between 10% and 20%. There were many problems with regard to cerebral ischemia. To reduce ischemic complications due to proximal vessel occlusion, collateral flow is provided via several types of bypass surgery [4, 5, 8, 12].

Retrograde recanalization of the internal carotid artery can be induced by backflow of the ophthalmic artery, posterior communicating artery and bypass arteries. Retrograde recanalization is thought to be the cause of aneurysmal enlargement.

Antegrade recanalization of the internal carotid artery can be induced by the collateral pathway between the internal and external carotid arteries, for example, the capsular artery, meningohypophyseal artery, inferior cavernous sinus artery, Vidian artery and caroticotympanic artery [1, 6]. The petrous ICA gives rise to two arterial branches: the caroticotympanic and Vidian arteries. The caroticotympanic artery arises from the genu of the petrous ICA and supplies the middle ear cavity. The Vidian artery, identifiable in adults, is an inconstant branch that arises from the horizontal petrous ICA in approximately 30% of temporal bone dissections [10]. This artery anastomoses with the ECA via a branch of the accessory meningeal, pterygovaginal and ascending pharyngeal arteries. The meningohypophyseal artery arises laterally to the dorsum sellae at or just before the apex of the first curve of the intracavernous carotid, where it turns forward after leaving the foramen lacerum. It is approximately the same size as the ophthalmic artery. The inferior cavernous sinus artery, also called the inferolateral trunk, arises from the lateral side of the midportion of the horizontal segment of the intracavernous carotid artery approximately 5–8 mm distal to the origin of the meningohypophyseal trunk [11]. The antegrade recanalization is thought to be the cause of artery-to-artery embolism. We think the antegrade recanalization is more dangerous than the retrograde recanalization of the ICA.

Conclusion

Based on our experience, as late recanalization of the aneurysm occurs in some patients with an ECA-ICA collateral pathway, we recommend that intraoperative angiography should be performed to detect the ECA-ICA collateral pathway in proximal ligation of the ICA. In proximal ligation for extradural ICA aneurysms, the ECA-ICA collateral pathway should be considered. If the DSA shows filling of the ICA after ligation, PAO using detachable coils is recommended.

Disclosure The authors have no personal financial or institutional interest in any of the drugs, materials, or devices described in this article.

Conflict of interest statement We declare that we have no conflict of interest.

References

1. Allen JW, Alastra AJ, Nelson PK (2005) Proximal intracranial internal carotid artery branches: prevalence and importance for balloon occlusion test. J Neurosurg 102(1):45–52
2. Dolenc V (1983) Direct microsurgical repair of intracavernous vascular lesions. J Neurosurg 58(6):824–831
3. Field M, Jungreis CA, Chengelis N, Kromer H, Kirby L, Yonas H (2003) Symptomatic cavernous sinus aneurysms: management and outcome after carotid occlusion and selective cerebral revascularization. Am J Neuroradiol 24(6):1200–1207
4. Gelber BR, Sundt TM Jr (1980) Treatment of intracavernous and giant carotid aneurysms by combined internal carotid ligation and extra- to intracranial bypass. J Neurosurg 52(1):1–10
5. Inoue T, Matsushima T, Fujii K, Hisada K, Fukui M (1996) Surgical treatment of intracavernous internal carotid artery aneurysm: bypass surgery. Jpn J Neurosurg (Tokyo) 5:188–193
6. Kagawa K, Shimizu H, Matsumoto Y, Watanabe M, Tominaga T (2007) Rapid revascularization after therapeutic parent artery occlusion for a large intracavernous carotid artery aneurysm. Neurol Med Chir (Tokyo) 47(12):559–563
7. Kai Y, Hamada J, Morioka M, Yano S, Mizuno T, Kuroda J, Todaka T, Takeshima H, Kuratsu J (2007) Treatment strategy for giant aneurysms in the cavernous portion of the internal carotid artery. Surg Neurol 67(2):148–155
8. Linskey ME, Jungreis CA, Yonas H, Hirsch WL Jr, Sekhar LN, Horton JA, Janosky JE (1994) Stroke risk after abrupt internal

carotid artery sacrifice: accuracy of preoperative assessment with balloon test occlusion and stable xenon-enhanced CT. Am J Neuroradiol 15(5):829–843
9. Niiro M, Shimozuru T, Nakamura K, Kadota K, Kuratsu J (2000) Long-term follow-up study of patients with cavernous sinus aneurysm treated by proximal occlusion. Neurol Med Chir (Tokyo) 40(2):88–96
10. Paullus WS, Pait TG, Rhoton AI Jr (1977) Microsurgical exposure of the petrous portion of the carotid artery. J Neurosurg 47(5):713–726
11. Rhoton AL Jr (2002) The cavernous sinus, the cavernous venous plexus, and the carotid collar. Neurosurgery 51(4 Suppl):S375–S410
12. Roski RA, Spetzler RF, Nulsen FE (1981) Late complication of carotid ligation in the treatment of intracranial aneurysms. J Neurosurg 54:583–587

Aneurysms of the Posterior Cerebral Artery and Approach Selection in Their Microsurgical Treatment: Emphasis on the Approaches: SAHEA and SCTTA

Yasuhiro Yonekawa, P. Roth, J. Fandino, and H. Landolt

Abstract Aneurysms of the posterior cerebral artery (PCA) are infrequent and located in the central depth of the brain. Hence their optimal microsurgical management has not been discussed systematically, as institutions and/or neurosurgeons have only limited experience. The purpose of this communication is to report our considerations on this topic with emphasis on the selection of approaches by reviewing our 20 consecutive cases of PCA aneurysms out of more than 1,000 aneurysm patients seen over the past 15 years. Although the subtemporal approach appears to be prevalent in the literature, in our series we applied the pterional approach with or without selective extradural anterior clinoidectomy (SEAC) for P1, P1-P2 aneurysms, and either a selective amygdalohippocampectomy approach (SAHEA) or supracerebellar transtentorial approach (SCTTA) for P2 and P2-P3 aneurysms. Construction of an extracranial-intracranial EC-IC bypass, when necessary, in conjunction with parent artery occlusion or with trapping of aneurysms was adapted to selected approaches.

Keywords PCA aneurysm · Approach · Selective amygdalohippocampectomy approach (SAHEA) · Supracerebellar transtentorial approach (SCTTA) · Extracranial-intracranial (EC-IC) bypass

Y. Yonekawa (✉)
Neurochirurgie FMH, University of Zürich,
Haldenbachstrasse 18, 8091 Zürich, Switzerland,
Klinik im Park, Zürich, Switzerland and
Department of Neurosurgery, Kantonsspital Aarau, Aarau, Switzerland
e-mail: yonekawa@usz.ch

P. Roth, J. Fandino, and H. Landolt
Department of Neurosurgery, Kantonsspital Aarau, Aarau, Switzerland

Introduction

Aneurysms of the posterior cerebral artery (PCA) are infrequent [3, 8] and located in the center of the brain, covered by the brain and bony structures of the skull. Accordingly, reports on this topic are rare, although Drake et al. published a pioneering report on 125 patients (59 non-giant aneurysms and 66 giant aneurysms) by using the subtemporal approach [3]. This approach, even in recent reports [13, 27], is considered standard, especially for aneurysms of the P2 segment. Only a limited number of authors have studied the approaches used to treat aneurysms of the PCA. Such approaches include, for example, the pterional approach for P1, P1-2 aneurysms, the subtemporal approach for P2 aneurysms and transoccipital interhemispheric approach for P3 aneurysms, as described by Yasargil in reviewing his 11 cases [19], or the transzygomatic approach described by Gerber et al. reporting on 2 cases [4]. We believe that appropriate approaches should take into account the locations of aneurysms and the swollen state of the brain in the acute stage of subarachnoid hemorrhage (SAH) with or without intracerebral hematoma (ICH) or intraventricular hematoma (IVH). This is why we are of the opinion that the selective amygdalohippocampectomy approach (SAHEA) [20, 24] or supracerebellar transtentorial approach (SCTTA) [23] should be considered for aneurysms of the P2, P2-P3 segment, especially in the acute stage of SAH.

Patients and Results

Twenty consecutive patients harboring PCA aneurysms were identified from more than 1,000 aneurysm patients and were analyzed according to the location of the PCA segment – P1, P2, or P3 with its periphery – and the approaches to the aneurysms. Clinical details of the patients are listed in Table 1. The female/male ratio was 3/1, and the average age was 44.6 ± 13.6 years. There were 15 ruptured aneurysms vassociated with intracerebral hematoma ICH and/

DOI: 10.1007/978-3-7091-0661-7_15,

Table 1

		Seg.	Side size	Grade		Approaches procedures	Procedures	GOS
1. HU	M 50	rupt P3	rt 1 cm	IV/V	IVH ICHH	Transoccip Trapping		4
2. SU	M 31	n rupt P2	rt 2.5 cm	O		SAHEA	STA-PCA bypass	5
3. BL	F 41	rupt P2-3	rt 4 cm	IV/V	IVH	SAHEA P2 occl		1
4. ZM	F 57	rup P2-3	rt 5 mm	III	ICH	SCTT		5
5. CA	F 62	n.rup P1	rt 3 mm	III		SAHEA P2 occl		5
6. BN	F 53	inc P1	lt 6 mm	O		Pter		5
7. CA	F 33	rup P1	lt 1 cm	IV	Dissection	Pter+SEAC BA occl		1
8. GA	F 51	n.rup P1	lt 3 mm	O		Pter		5
9. HP	F 53	rup P1	lt 1.5 cm	IV/V		Pter		3
10. BM	M 18	inc P1	lt 2 mm	O		Pter Coating		5
11. RL	F 65	rup P2	rt 3 cm	III		SCTTA P2 occl		4
12. JK	M 44	n rup P2	lt 2 cm	Symp		SCTTA P2 occl.	STA-PCA bypass	5
13. SH	F 68	rup P1-P2	lt 1.5 cm	IV/V		Pter		1
14. PR	F 33	rup P1-P2	lt 2.5 cm	IV/V		Pter-SEAC		4
15. HJ	F 40	rup P1	lt 1 cm	I	Dissection	Pter+SEAC		5
16. HA	M 17	rup P2-P3	lt 1 cm	IV/V	IVH	SCTTA		1
17. BJ	F 47	n rupP2-P3	lt 4 mm	III		SCTTA		5
18. PL	F 38	rup P2/P3	rt 1 mm	III		SAHEA P2 occl		5
19. PC	F 45	rup P1	lt 1.5 cm	II		SCTTA	OA-PCA bypass	4
20. UD	F 35	rup P2	rt 7 mm	I	Dissection	SAHEA		2

or intraventricular hematoma IVH (25%). These aneurysms were located in segments P1 (8, 40%), P1-P2 (2,10%), P2 (4, 20%), P2-P3 (5, 25%) and P3 and its periphery (1, 5%). The patients underwent the following surgical approaches: pterional [with or without selective anterior clinoidectomy (SEAC) (8, 40%), SCTTA (6, 30%), SAHEA (5, 25%) and transoccipital (1, 5%)]. The following surgical treatments were performed: neck clipping (9, 45%), trapping (3, 15%), parent artery occlusion (4, 20%), coating (2, 10%), endovascular coiling (1, 5%) and aneurysmorrhaphy (1, 5%). Extracranial-intracranial (EC-IC) bypass to the distal part of the PCA was performed in three patients at the time of parent artery occlusion and aneurysm trapping. The Glasgow Outcome Scale (GOS) score [7] 6 months postoperatively was: 4–5 (13, 65%), 3 (2, 10%), 2(1, 5%) and 1 (4, 20%).

Representative Cases

Case 2 (Fig. 1)

This 31-year-old male had been suffering from frequent hemicrania irradiating into the right eye for 3 years. Three months prior to initial presentation, he had experienced a severe headache for 5 days, leading to magnetic resonance imaging (MRI)

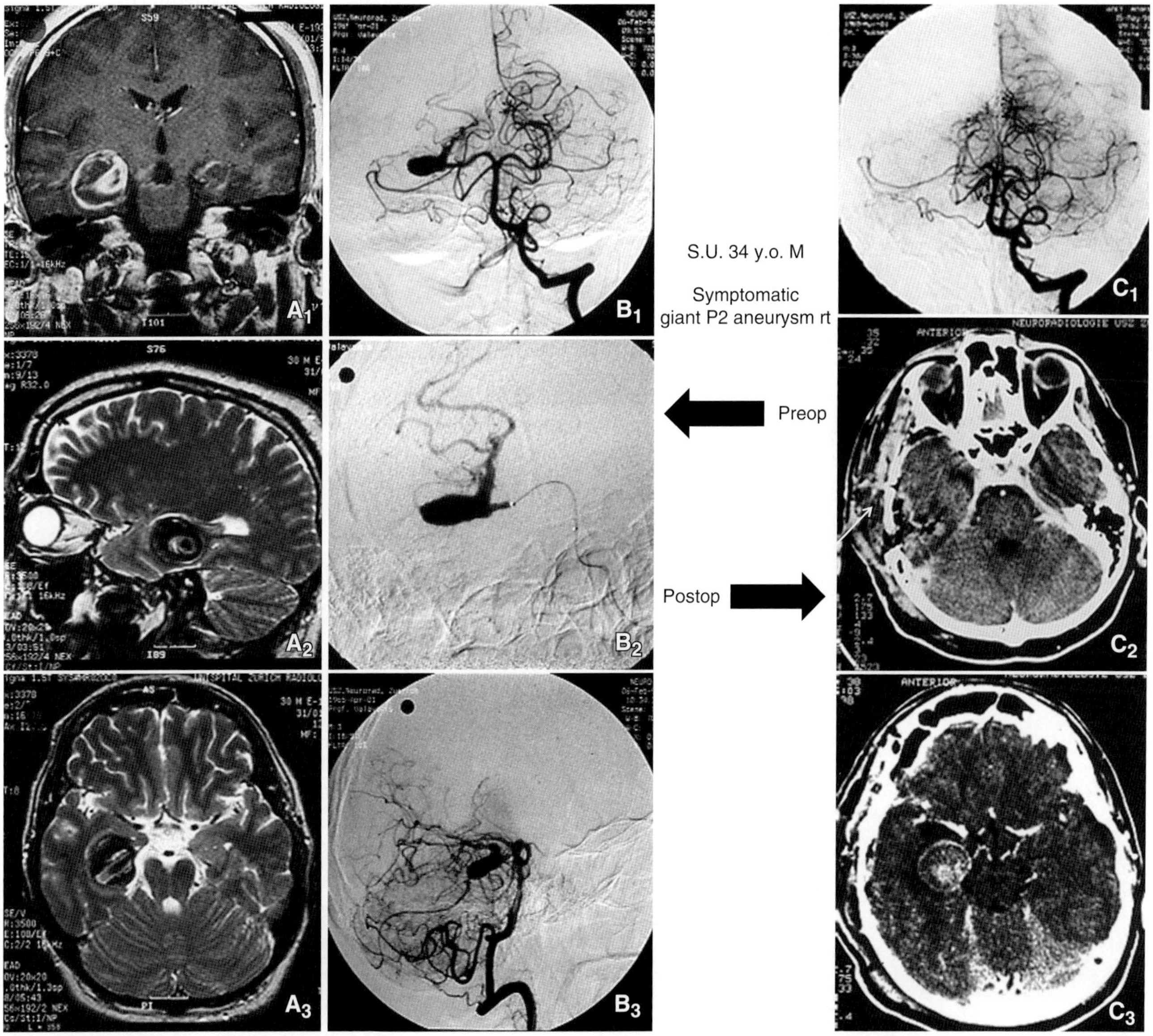

Fig. 1 Case 2: A 31-year-old male with mostly thrombosed giant aneurysm at the right P2-P3 segment junction. A1-A3: Preoperative MRIs show a mostly thrombosed giant aneurysm at the right hippocampal-parahippocampal region, B1-B3: DSA confirms the aneurysm. C1: Follow-up angiography shows no visualization of the aneurysm and no filling of distal segments of the right PCA. Patency of the STA-PCA bypass is shown with an *arrow* on the postoperative CT scan (C2). Postoperative CTs display no infarction at the right temporo-occipital region in spite of proximal ligation of the PCA at the P2 segment

examination, which disclosed a mostly thrombosed giant aneurysm of 2.5 cm at the right P2-P3 segment junction. The patient reported neither epileptic seizures nor visual field disturbance. The aneurysm was confirmed by digital subtraction angiography (DSA). During the DSA procedure, a balloon occlusion test (BOT) at the right P2 segment was performed, and the patient experienced a remarkable reduction in the severity of the headache, but had some visual field disturbance simultaneously. This giant aneurysm was treated by proximal occlusion at the P2 segment using SAHEA plus extracranial-intracranial (EC-IC) bypass between the superficial temporal artery (STA) and a temporobasal cortical branch of the PCA. The patient recovered well from the procedure without any neurological deficits and had a GOS score of 5 at the postoperative 6-month follow-up.

Comment

In this case a combination of proximal parent artery ligation plus EC-IC bypass was effective after the non-tolerated BOT. Exposure of the giant aneurysm and P2 portion could be performed using SAHEA. Neck clipping proved to be impossible because of the size of the aneurysm and its atheromatous plaque around the neck. Proximal ligation at the P2 segment could be done after construction of an EC-IC bypass at the posterobasal corner of the same craniotomy.

Case 11 (Fig. 2)

This 65-year-old female had been suffering from nuchal headache and nausea for 2 days. Her past history included an operation for a ruptured aneurysm of the anterior communicating artery (AcomA) 7 years prior to her current clinical presentation. Her Glasgow Coma Scale (GCS) score [14] was 13 with remarkable confusion at the time of hospitalization. A computed tomography (CT) scan revealed an ICH at the right basal ganglia with a presumably thrombosed giant aneurysm. After DSA confirmation of an aneurysm of 3 cm in diameter at the right P2 segment, the aneurysm was exposed, and proximal ligation was performed at the right P2 segment with SCTTA accompanied by the removal of a peri-aneurysmal ICH. Although simultaneous construction of an

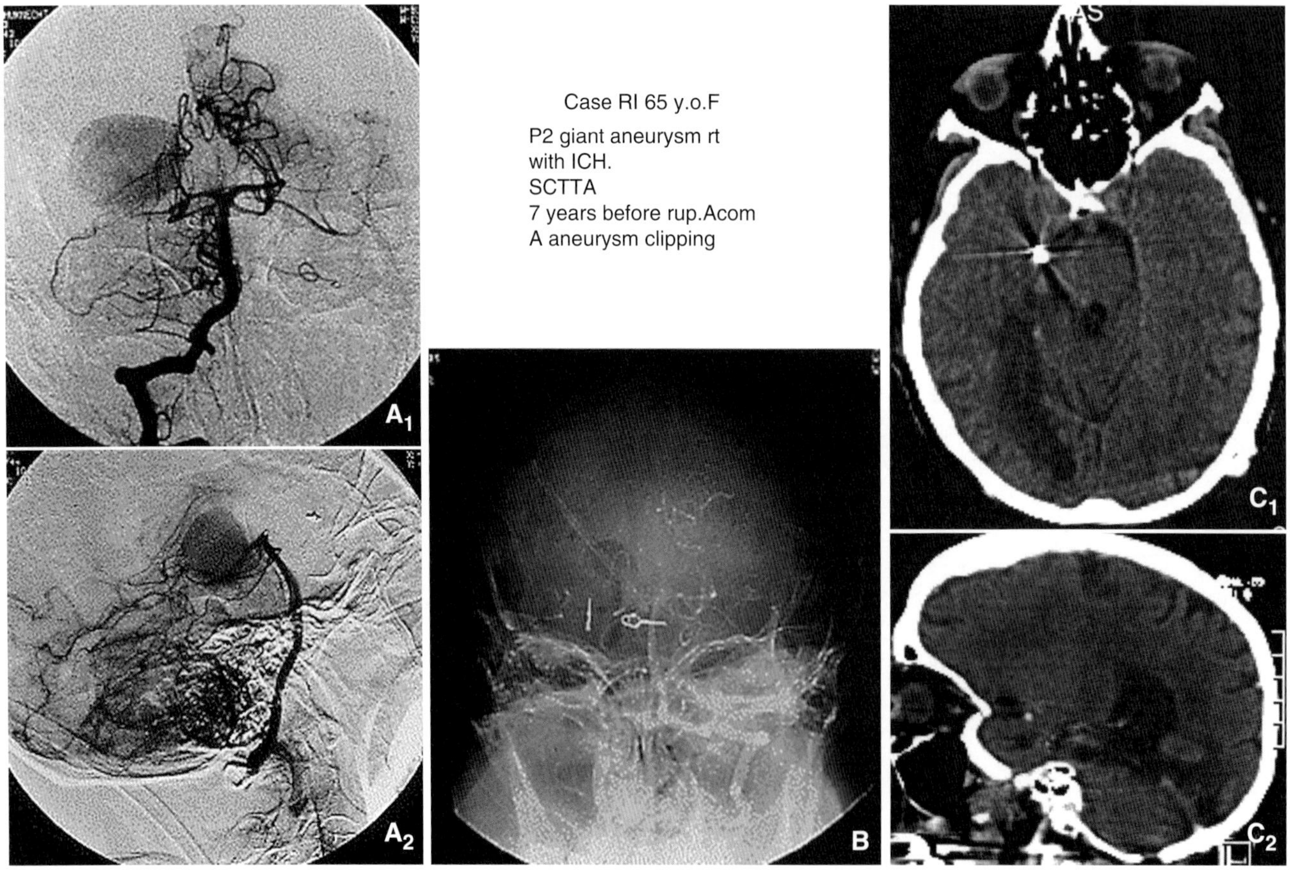

Fig. 2 Case 11: A 65-year-old female with ruptured giant aneurysm at the P2 segment with ICH. A1-A2: Preoperative DSA shows a giant aneurysm at the P2 segment. B: Follow-up angiography displays no visualization of the aneurysm, with two clips at the P2 segment for parent artery occlusion and at the AcomA (see text). C1, C2: Follow-up CT scan 9 years later shows partial infarction at the right P3 territory and disappearance of the aneurysm at the right hippocampo-parahippocampal region

EC-IC bypass was planned in the same approach, it failed because of an extremely atheromatous donor occipital artery (OA). Intraoperative cerebral blood flow (CBF) monitoring with a Peltier stack displayed a gradual but sufficient recovery at the distal part of the cortex on P2 proximal ligation, so that sufficient collateral supply to the distal part of the PCA was presumed. The patient recovered well from the procedure, but with partial hemianopsia because of a partial infarction of the P3 segment. Insertion of a ventriculo-peritoneal shunt followed because of communicating hydrocephalus. The GOS score was 4 at the 6-month follow-up.

Comment

This is a representative case in which aneurysm exposure at the P2 portion can be performed with SCTTA in the acute stage of bleeding. Although simultaneous EC-IC bypass construction failed because of the diseased OA, this could normally have been performed using the same approach [22, 23]. Also, this case shows that intraoperative CBF monitoring can help determine the definitive procedures: clipping, and proximal ligation with or without EC-IC bypass in case of lacking a systematic preoperative BOT [10, 21].

Case 20 (Fig. 3)

This 35-year-old female had suffered SAH 2 months prior to her current clinical presentation. She recovered well, and a neuroradiological examination disclosed a dissecting aneurysm of 7 mm at the right P2 segment. She underwent surgery in the chronic stage with a GCS score of 15. Access to the aneurysm was successful using SAHEA with exposure of the whole P2 segment, but neck clipping was complicated by premature rupture, so that an aneurysmorrhaphy had to be performed with continuous suture using a 9–0 monofilament after removal of a considerable portion of the aneurysm.

Case UR 35 y.o. F P2 dissection aneurysm

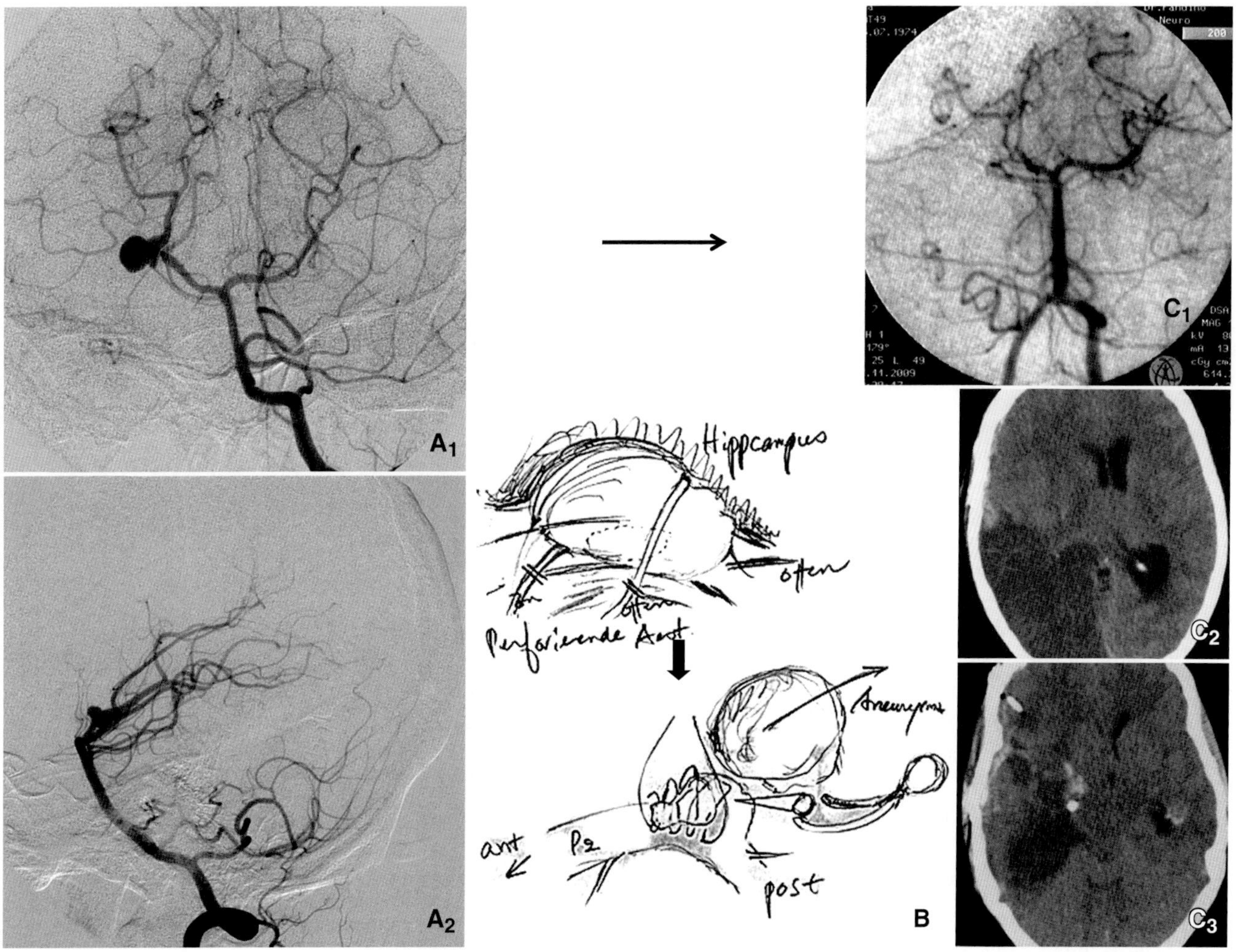

Fig. 3 Case 29: A 35-year-old female with ruptured dissecting aneurysm at the P2 segment. A1 and A2 reveal the aneurysm indicating partly "string and beads sign" on DSA. B: Surgeon's sketch showing the aneurysm removal and aneurysmorrhaphy, as the pre-ruptured aneurysm turned out to be unclippable. C1 displays intraoperative angiography showing the patency of the right P2 segment after aneurysmorrhaphy. C2-C3 CT scans several days after surgery indicate an extensive infarction of PCA and part of the MCA territory

Intraoperative angiography showed good patency of the segment. The patient was awake directly after surgery with slight hemiparesis, which is observed quite often after surgery with this approach for SAHE [24]. However, a few days later the paresis became worse and was accompanied by altered consciousness. A follow-up CT scan displayed an extensive infarction at the territory of the PCA as well as partly at the MCA territory. In spite of the best available treatment for ischemic edema and rehabilitation, the patient's GOS score remained 2–3 at the 6-month follow-up.

Comment

This is a typical case of a complication associated with the clipping procedure for dissecting aneurysms – namely, unclippable premature rupture – necessitating aneurysmorrhaphy. Although patency was confirmed by intraoperative angiography, the site of aneurysmorrhaphy must have closed with thrombus formation, followed by its propagation over the P2-P3 junction in a few days. Retraction of the MCA at the time of SAHEA must have also caused an insufficient postoperative collateral supply from the MCA territory to the diseased PCA territory. If the SCTTA approach had been taken instead of SAHEA, optimal clipping could have been performed or at least clean proximal ligation or trapping would have been possible, so that the P2-P3 junction closure because of thrombus propagation could have been prevented, resulting in better collateral supply at the distal territory of the PCA. Also presumably insufficient collateral supply from the MCA to the PCA territory due to SAHEA could have been prevented by using SCTTA.

Discussion

The following characteristics of PCA aneurysms can be summarized on the basis of hitherto published reports and the authors' observations:

1. Infrequency – PCA aneurysms represent less than a few percent of all aneurysms [6, 8, 13, 26].
2. Good collateralization of the PCA territory, but a significant percentage of ischemic complications occur in connection with proximal parent artery occlusion, e.g., up to 17% of patients suffer from new visual field deficits; hence, the need for an EC-IC bypass combination has been discussed [2, 3, 13, 16].
3. Up to 50% of all PCA aneurysms are large or giant aneurysms [3, 13].

The results of our series coincide well with those of other previous reports. These characteristics and the limited experience neurosurgeons and/or interventional neuroradiologists make the treatment complex even also with combination of these techniques. Especially the management of the very rare dissecting aneurysms of the PCA deserves further evaluation for treatment standardization, also in light of the technical development of endovascular surgery [1, 12, 15].

Regarding approaches for microsurgical treatment, the subtemporal approach pioneered by Drake has been predominant, even in recent reports [3, 13, 27], although the pterional approach has gained a solid position in the microsurgical management of aneurysms at the P1 and P1-P2 segments [6, 11, 13]. In our series with 15 cases of SAH in its acute stage (75%), the subtemporal approach was applied in none of the cases. The standard pterional approach opening the proximal sylvian fissure was applied for the P1 and P1-P2 aneuryms, and SEAC was added in three cases of large or giant aneurysms to make the complicated microsurgical procedure in a deep location smoother [25]. The SAHEA is a kind of pterional approach, but differs from it in that the distal sylvian fissure is opened as well as the choroidal fissure after reaching the temporal horn by having access through the temporal stem with a small cortical incision (around 1.5 cm) at the sulcus circularis insulae [20, 24]. This approach allows dissection of the whole stretch of the P2 segment from its origin to the P2-P3 junction, even when the brain is swollen because of SAH, and with or without hematoma during slight to moderate retraction of the cortical incision (Fig. 4). CSF can be drained by opening the basal cistern, the lamina terminalis and the temporal horn in the same craniotomy,

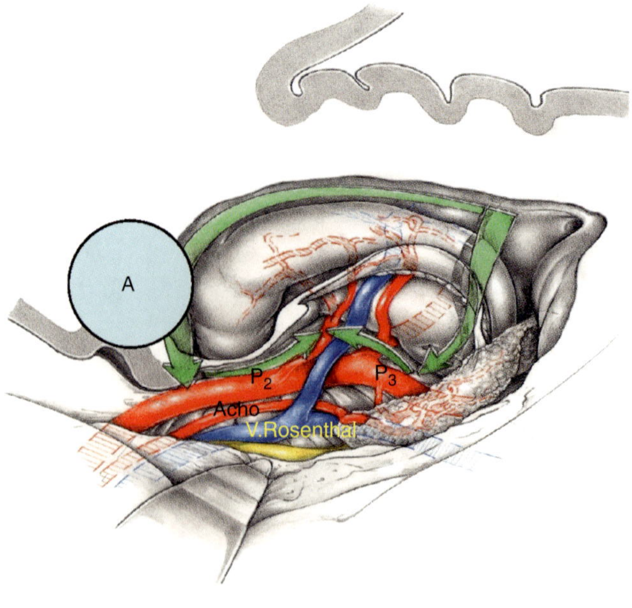

Fig. 4 SAHEA showing structures after opening the choroidal fissure for dissection of the PCA. *A*: amygdala, *Acho*: anterior choroidal artery. *Green arrows* are for the selective amygdalohippocampectomy [24]

enabling brain slackness. If an EC-IC bypass is needed, it can be combined with the above-mentioned procedure for aneurysms by using the STA as a donor and a cortical branch of the PCA at the posterior temporobasal corner of the craniotomy, as was done in the above-mentioned case 2.

As for SCTTA in the sitting position, used in six cases in this series, we reported on the topic in 2001 for lesions of posterior temporomedial structures, in which the microsurgical management of a ruptured P2 giant aneurysm and of a P2-P3 junction aneurysm with ICH and occipital artery OA-PCA bypass were also included [23]. The PCA can be followed proximally as far as its crossing point with the third nerve, so that every procedure for microsurgical aneurysm management is possible without compromising the gyrus parahippocampalis, even when the brain is swollen because of SAH. If an EC-IC bypass is needed, this can be performed in the same craniotomy session using the OA, auriculotemporal artery ATA or even the STA as donor and the cortical branch of the PCA as recipient at the temporo-medial cortex. This bypass procedure was combined with an aneurysm coiling procedure for case 19. A comparison between SAHEA, the transtemporal approach [17], subtemporal approach and SCTTA is presented in Fig. 5 by an artist's drawing.

Successful surgical and endovascular occlusion of unclippable PCA aneurysms has been reported by several authors, and this was ascribed to relatively good collateralization to the distal territory of the occluded PCA [3, 5, 18]. Although the bypass procedure in combination with proximal ligation

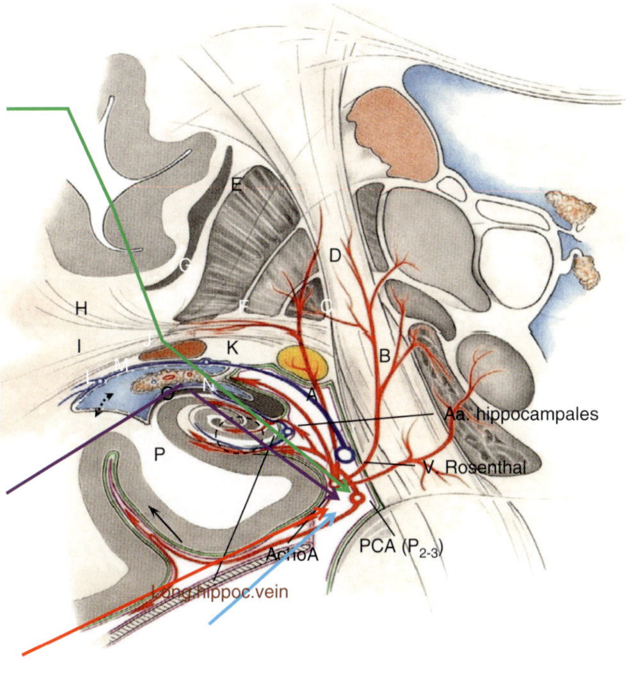

Fig. 5 Four illustrative accesses to the PCA (P2-P2-3 segment) are shown: *green arrow*: SAHEA; *violet arrow*: transtemporal approach [17]; *brown arrow*: subtemporal approach; *blue arrow*: SCTTA

of the parent artery or with aneurysm trapping is considered to be effective, extensive infarction of the PCA territory in spite of a patent EC-IC bypass has been reported by Murai et al. [9]. Although they attributed this complication to insufficient postoperative management against ischemia, propagation of thrombus over the P2-P3 junction is also considered to be responsible as in our case of aneurysmorrhaphy. An intentional occlusion of the distal part of the aneurysm just prior to the P2-P3 junction (and not only proximal occlusion) could have prevented this complication as collateral circulation between the distal P3 segment would have remained intact.

Conclusion

Infrequent PCA aneurysms necessitate deliberate treatment planning, especially with regard to approach selection based on the aneurysm's location, size and associated hematomas. The pterional approach with or without SEAC is suitable for P1 and P1-P2 aneurysms, while the SAHEA in the supine position or the SCTTA in the sitting position should be considered for P2 and/or P2-P3 aneurysms. These can be performed not only for swollen brains in the acute stage of SAH, but also when an EC-IC bypass is required by the findings of a BOT.

Acknowledgment The authors are indebted to Ms. R. Frick and Ms. H. Job for their technical and secretarial assistance, and Dr. N. Khan for English correction.

Conflict of interest statement We declare that we have no conflict of interest.

References

1. Berger MSWC (1984) Intracranial dissecting aneurysms of the posterior circulation. Report of six cases and review of the literature. J Neurosurg 61:882–894
2. Chang HS, Fukushima T, Takakura K et al (1986) Aneurysms of the posterior cerebral artery: report of 10 cases. Neurosurgery 19: 1006–1011
3. Drake C, Peerless SJ, Hernesniemi JA (1996) Non-giant aneurysms of the posterior cerebral artery: 59 patients. Giant posterior cerebral aneurysms: 66 patients. In: Drake C, Peerless SJ, Hernesniemi JA (eds) Surgery of vertebrobasilar aneurysms. Springer, Wien, pp 221–248
4. Gerber C, Neil-Dwyer G, Barrie E (1993) An alternative surgical approach to aneurysms of the posterior cerebral artery. Neurosurgery 32:928–931
5. Hallacq P, Piotin M, Moret J (2002) Endovascular occlusion of the posterior cerebral artery for the treatment of P2 segment aneurysms: retrospective review of a 10-year series. Am J Neuroradiol 23: 1128–1136

6. Honda M, Tsutsumi K, Yokoyama H et al (2004) Aneurysms of the posterior cerebral artery: retrospective review of surgical treatment. Neurol Med Chir (Tokyo) 44:164–169
7. Jennet B, Bond M (1975) Assessment of outcome after severe brain damage. A practical scale. Lancet 1:480–484
8. Locksley H (1966) Report on the cooperative study of intracranial aneurysms and subarachnoid hemorrhage. Section 5, part 1. Natural history of subarachnoid hemorrhage, intracranial aneurysms and arteriovenous malformations. Based on 6368 cases in the cooperative study. J Neurosurg 25:219–239
9. Murai Y, Adachi K, Yoshida Y et al (2010) Failure of combined treatment for the thrombosed posterior cerebral artery aneurysm. Surg Cereb Stroke (Jpn) 38:52–56
10. Ogata N, Fournier Y, Imhof HG, Yonakeawa Y (1996) Thermal diffusion blood flow monitoring during aneurysm surgery. Acta Neurochir 138:726–731
11. Sakata S, Fujii K, Matsushima T et al (1993) Aneurysm of the posterior cerebral artery: report of eleven cases – surgical approaches and procedures. Neurosurgery 32:163–168, discussion 167–168
12. Shinno K, Nagahiro S, Nishide S (2010) A clinical analysis of posterior cerebral artery dissection with special reference to management and outcome. Surg Cereb Stroke (Jpn) 38:95–100
13. Taylor CL, Kopitonik TA, Samson D, Purdy PD (2003) Treatment and outcome in 30 patients with posterior cerebral artery aneurysms. J Neurosurg 99:15–22
14. Teasdale G, Jennet B (1974) Assessment of coma and impaired consciousness. A practical scale. Lancet 2:81–84
15. Tsukahara T, Minematsu K (2010) Overview of spontaneous cervicocephalic arterial dissection in Japan. Acta Neurochir Suppl 107:35–40
16. Vishteh AG, Smith KA, McDougall CG, Spetzler RF (1998) Distal posterior cerebral artery vascularization in multimodality management of complex peripheral posterior cerebral artery aneurysms: technical case report. Neurosurgery 43:166–170
17. Wu A, Chang SW, Desmukh P et al (2010) Through the choroidal fissure: a quantitative anatomic comparison of 2 incisions and trajectories (Transsylvian transchoroidal and lateral transtemporal). Neurosurgery 66:221–228, discussion 228–229
18. Yamashita K, Taki W, Nishi S et al (1992) Treatment of unclippable giant posterior cerebral artery aneurysms with detachable balloons – report of three cases. Neurol Med Chir (Tokyo) 32:679–683
19. Yasargil MG (1984) Vertebrobasilar aneurysms. In: Yasargil MG (ed) Microneurosurgery, vol 2. Georg Thieme, Stuttgart, pp 232–295
20. Yasargil MG, Krayenbühl N, Roth P et al (2010) The selective amygdalohippocampectomy for intractable limbic seizures. J Neurosurg 112:168–185
21. Yonekawa Y (2009) Brain vascularization by extracranial-intracranial arterial bypass. In: Sindou M (ed) Practical hand book of neurosurgery, vol Vol1. Springer, Wien, pp 355–381
22. Yonekawa Y (2010) Posterior circulation EC-IC bypass via supracerebellar transtentorial SCTT approach applied in a young patient with congenial multiple occlusive cerebrovascular anomalies. Acta Neurochir Suppl 17:89–93
23. Yonekawa Y, Imhof HG, Taub E et al (2001) Supracerebellar transtentorial approach for posterior temporomedial structures. J Neurosurg 94:339–345
24. Yonekawa Y, Leblebicioglu-Könu D, Strommer K, Wieser G (1996) Selective amygdalohippocampectomy according to Yasargil-Wieser for intractable epilepsy. Neurosurgeons 15:184–191
25. Yonekawa Y, Ogata N, Imhof HG et al (1997) Selective extradural anterior clinoidectomy for supra- and parasellar processes. J Neurosurg 87:636–642
26. Zeal A, Rhoton AJr (1978) Microsurgical anatomy of the posterior cerebral artery. J Neurosurg 48:534–559
27. Zhitao J, Yibao W, Anhua W et al (2010) Microsurgical subtemporal approach to aneurysms on the P2 segment of the posterior cerebral artery. Neurol India 58:242–247

Resistant Vasospasm in Subarachnoid Hemorrhage Treated with Continuous Intraarterial Nimodipine Infusion

A. Doukas*, A.K. Petridis*, H. Barth, O. Jansen, H. Maslehaty, and H.M. Mehdorn

Abstract Cerebral vasospasm complicating aneurysmal subarachnoid hemorrhage is a well-known medical entity. The delayed ischemic neurological deficits (DIND) as a result of vasospasm remain the main cause of morbidity among patients who manage to survive this severe disease pattern. When the traditional treatment options, either medical or interventional, fail to reverse vasospasm, continuous intraarterial infusion of nimodipine through catheters directly into the spastic arteries presents a promising treatment modality. Of 73 patients with aneurysmal subarachnoid hemorrhage between 2008 and 2009, a total of 27 had Hunt and Hess grades of 4 and 5. Fifteen percent of them showed refractory vasospasms and were treated with continuous nimodipine infusion via catheters in both internal carotid arteries. We present the method's indications and possible complications.

Keywords Aneurysm · Subarachnoid hemorrhage · Vasospasm · Intraarterial continuous nimodipine

Abbreviation

ICA Internal carotid artery

Introduction

Cerebral vasospasm complicating aneurysmal subarachnoid hemorrhage is a well-known medical entity. The first published report came from Ecker and Riemenschneider in 1951 and 1953 [7, 8]. In the subsequent years, scientists tried to study vasospasm in animal models [31], while the first announcement of vasospasm-induced cerebral infarction appeared 2 years later by Simeone and Trepper [26]. Since then, many treatment methods have been proposed and applied. Nevertheless, delayed ischemic neurological deficits (DIND) as a result of vasospasm, occurring in approximately 30% of the patients, remain the main cause of morbidity [12, 29]. The peak frequency of vasospasm usually starts on days 3–5 of subarachnoid hemorrhage (SAH). It exhibits maximal narrowing of the arterial lumen during days 5–14, and slowly resolves until 4 weeks after the initial incident [18]. We herein describe the administration of continuous nimodipine infusion via catheters in the ICAs until, if possible, vasospasms resolve.

Materials and Methods

Between 2008 and 2009, 73 patients with SAH were treated in our clinic. The mean Hunt and Hess score was 3.07. In 56 of the patients the etiology of SAH was rupture of intracranial aneurysms; in 17 patients no etiology could be found. Thirty-one aneurysms were clipped, 23 were coiled, and two both clipped and coiled. Twenty-seven of the patients had poor Hunt and Hess grades after subarachnoid hemorrhage (4 and 5), and of those who developed refractory vasospasm, 15% received continuous intraarterial nimodipine infusion via catheters in both ICAs. All patients were treated in our neurosurgical intensive care unit. The intubated and sedated patients received continuous monitoring of the intracranial pressure and cerebral mean oxygen pressure, and had external ventricular drain.

A. Doukas (✉), A.K. Petridis, H. Barth, H. Maslehaty, and H.M. Mehdorn
Department of Neurosurgery, University Hospital of Schleswig-Holstein, Campus Kiel, Schittenhelmstrasse 10, 24105 Kiel, Germany
e-mail: axlpam@yahoo.com

O. Jansen
Institute of Neuroradiology, University Hospital of Schleswig-Holstein, Campus Kiel, Schittenhelmstrasse 10, 24105 Kiel, Germany

*A. Doukas, A.K. Petridis contributed equally to this work

DOI: 10.1007/978-3-7091-0661-7_16,

Selection Criteria for the Administration of Continuous Nimodipine Infusion

All patients with aneurysmal subarachnoid hemorrhage treated in our clinic received triple H therapy (hypervolemia, hypertension, and hemodilution) as well as nimodipine the moment they developed vasospasm. By stable clinical status or by normal perfusion CT findings, which were routinely carried out on the 3rd and 7th day after the onset of SAH, the therapy was continued with cerebral perfusion pressure (CPP) of over 100 mmHg.

Patients considered for continuous nimodipine infusion were chosen according to the following parameters: evidence of increased flow velocities via Doppler sonography (abnormal Gosling and Pourcelot indices) with impairment of the brain tissue perfusion in the perfusion CAT scan led to immediate angiography. Vasospastic vessels were dilated with balloon angioplasty (proximal vessels, i.e., M1, A1, P1) or with local nimodipine application. The patient came back to the intensive care unit where the Doppler examinations were continued. If the vasospasm(s) would not resolve completely or satisfactorily according to the aforementioned indices or if the patients clinically deteriorated, for those who were not intubated, we would decide to implant the catheters in both ICAs for continuous nimodipine infusion. The initial Hunt and Hess score or Fisher grade was not considered as a criterion for the administration of such a therapy, while all patients had a Hunt and Hess score of 3 or more and in the CAT scan Fisher grade of 3 or 4.

Patients and Methods

Of the patients admitted and treated in our department, four showed massive vasospasms after suffering an aneurysmal SAH and were treated by the aforementioned method. The vasospasms were documented via transcranial Doppler, and perfusion CAT scans were used for confirmation. Thereafter the patients were transferred to the neuroradiological institute, and a digital subtraction angiography with local dilatation of the spastic arteries with nimodipine was performed. In case of a positive response, that is, adequate vasodilatation, the catheters were left in both internal carotid arteries for continuous infusion of nimodipine. The decision whether to place the catheters in both ICAs or in only one was made according to the findings of the angiography, i.e., if vasospasms were on both sides or not.

The infusion scheme was as follows: 5 mg nimodipine were slowly administered via an infusion pump with 5 ml/h for each side.

On the following day, angiography as well as perfusion CAT scan was repeated (Fig. 1), and if the vasospasms had not resolved, the infusion was continued. Maximal duration of the infusion was 72 h.

Complications

In our small patient series we had one iatrogenic carotid dissection, which was treated with stent implantation. Other possible complications, which did however not occur in our

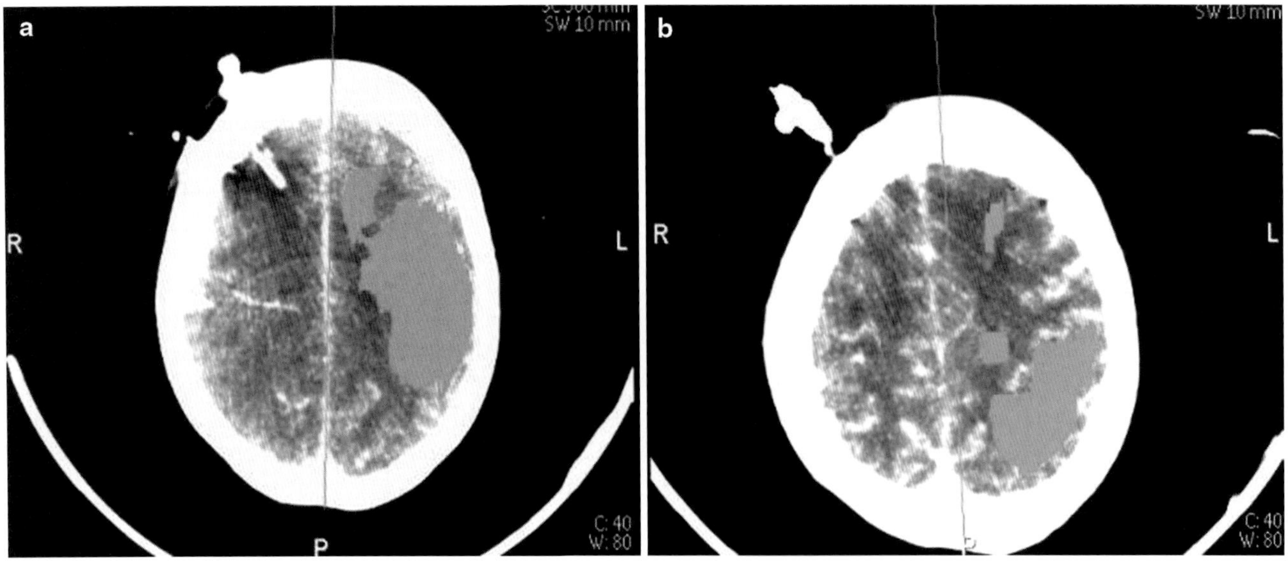

Fig. 1 Perfusion CAT scan before (**a**) and after (**b**) administration of intraarterial continuous nimodipine via both ICAs shows regression of tissue at risk in the MCA territory on the *left side*

patients, might be thromboembolism, significant lowering of the systemic blood pressure, occlusion or dislocation of the catheters and infections.

Discussion

Many therapeutic options have already been described. The use of oral nimodipine is commonly accepted, with proven efficacy in many studies, especially in a large retrospective study of Dorhout Mees et al., which included 3,361 patients [5]. Based on the same concept, another calcium channel antagonist, nicardipine, was used to prevent or treat vasospasm, but not with the same efficacy as nimodipine [1]. The use of statins was also presented as very promising. Vergouwen et al. and McGirt et al. in their recent report found no statistically significant difference in clinical outcome, vasospasm or delayed neurological deficit in patients treated with statins [20, 29], whereas Sillberg et al. showed that initiation of statin therapy after aneurysmal SAH significantly reduces the incidence of vasospasm, delayed ischemic deficits, and mortality [25]. Another treatment option that could be potentially beneficial against DIND and cerebral ischemia is magnesium sulfate. Currently, two large phase II trials are being conducted that will hopefully provide definite evidence whether magnesium treatment is beneficial in SAH patients, as could be shown in rats [6, 27, 28, 32, 33]. Veyna et al. already observed a trend towards a Glasgow Outcome Scale (GOS) score of 4 or 5, but this trend did not reach a statistically significant level [30].

Among the multiple treatment options regarding resistant vasospasm after aneurysmal SAH, intraarterial infusion of pharmacological agents has gained the attention of neurosurgeons and neuroradiologists. Eskridge et al. proposed the following criteria regarding endovascular treatment of restrictive vasospasm after SAH: (1) new onset of neurological deficit not due to other causes; (2) no evidence of cerebral infarction on the CT scan; (3) a persistent deficit not responding to triple H therapy (hypervolemia, hypertension, and hemodilution), and (4) angiographic evidence of vasospasm in a distribution explaining the neurological deficit. Newell et al. also indicated that balloon angioplasty should be considered as a safe treatment method with good results and low complication rates [10, 22]. Böker et al. reported three cases of subarachnoid hemorrhage and cerebral vasospasm treated with intraarterial nimodipine infusion for 90 min. Resolution of the spasms was demonstrated with angiography [3]. Sayama et al. [24] as well as Eddleman et al. [9] and other study groups [4, 13–16, 19, 21, 23] also reported on endovascular therapies for cerebral vasospasm including transluminal balloon angioplasty and intraarterial vasodilating agents such as nimodipine, nicardipine, verapamil, or milrinone. They observed that papaverine managed to dilate the spastic vessels but negatively influenced the intracranial pressure. They suggested that larger studies with intraarterial agents should be performed to achieve safer and more accurate results. Hänggi et al. as well as Kim et al. in their recent studies reported a positive response with the reduction of angiographic vasospasm after intraarterial nimodipine administration. Liu and co-workers stressed the efficacy of repeated papaverine infusions with a positive response of the diameter of the spastic vessels [11, 14].

Since the intraarterial infusion of nimodipine seems to resolve cerebral vasospasm and given the fact that its effect lasts for several hours, but then decreases and many patients require more than one intervention [2, 17], we tried to continuously administer nimodipine through catheters in both ICAs directly into the spastic arteries for 48–72 h controlling its effect with daily angiographic images, transcranial Doppler workups, and perfusion CAT scans.

Conclusions

We presented a new treatment method for aggressive vasospasm in patients with aneurysmal subarachnoid hemorrhage. In cases where conservative treatment cannot achieve resolution of the vasospasms and the eventually following ischemic deficits, and where intraarterial nimodipine administration shows good vessel widening, continuous nimodipine infusion via catheters in the ICA could be the last treatment chance. Through these catheters a daily angiographic study can be performed if needed. The number of patients we treated in this way was low, and more studies should be performed to show the method's efficacy. Further, when administration of this treatment method should be started as well as what should be the exact dose of nimodipine that can be given to maximize vasodilatation of the vessels with minimum adverse reactions still needs to be clarified.

Conflict of interest statement We declare that we have no conflict of interest.

References

1. Alaraj A, Charbel FT, Amin-Hanjani S (2009) Peri-operative measures for treatment and prevention of cerebral vasospasm following subarachnoid hemorrhage. Neurol Res 31(6):651–659, Epub Jan 7
2. Biondi A, Ricciardi GK, Puybasset L, Abdennour L, Longo M, Chiras J, Van Effenterre R (2004) Intra-arterial nimodipine for the treatment of symptomatic cerebral vasospasm after aneurysmal

subarachnoid hemorrhage: preliminary results. AJNR Am J Neuroradiol 25(6):1067–1076
3. Böker DK, Solymosi L, Wassmann H (1985) Immediate postangiographic intraarterial treatment of cerebral vasospasm after subarachnoid hemorrhage with nimodipine. Report on 3 cases. Neurochirurgia (Stuttg) 28(Suppl 1):118–120
4. Brisman JL, Eskridge JM, Newell DW (2006) Neurointerventional treatment of vasospasm. Neurol Res 28(7):769–776
5. Dorhout Mees SM, MASH-II study group (2008) Magnesium in aneurysmal subarachnoid hemorrhage (MASH II) phase III clinical trial MASH-II study group. Int J Stroke 3(1):63–65
6. Dorhout Mees SM, Rinkel GJ, Feigin VL, Algra A, van den Bergh WM, Vermeulen M, van Gijn J (2005) Calcium antagonists for aneurysmal subarachnoid haemorrhage. Cochrane Database Syst Rev (1):CD000277
7. Ecker A, Riemenschneider PA (1951) Arteriographic demonstration of spasm of the intracranial arteries, with special reference to saccular arterial aneurysms. J Neurosurg 8(6):660–667
8. Ecker A, Riemenschneider PA (1953) Arteriographic evidence of spasm in cerebral vascular disorders. Neurology 3(7):495–502
9. Eddleman CS, Hurley MC, Naidech AM, Batjer HH, Bendok BR (2009) Endovascular options in the treatment of delayed ischemic neurological deficits due to cerebral vasospasm. Neurosurg Focus 26(3):E6
10. Eskridge JM, Newell DW, Pendleton GA (1990) Transluminal angioplasty for treatment of vasospasm. Neurosurg Clin N Am 1(2):387–399
11. Hänggi D, Turowski B, Beseoglu K, Yong M, Steiger HJ (2008) Intra-arterial nimodipine for severe cerebral vasospasm after aneurysmal subarachnoid hemorrhage: influence on clinical course and cerebral perfusion. AJNR Am J Neuroradiol 29(6):1053–1060, Epub 2008
12. Hijdra A, Van Gijn J, Stefanko S, Van Dongen KJ, Vermeulen M, Van Crevel H (1986) Delayed cerebral ischemia after aneurysmal subarachnoid hemorrhage: clinicoanatomic correlations. Neurology 36(3):329–333
13. Hoh BL, Ogilvy CS (2005) Endovascular treatment of cerebral vasospasm: transluminal balloon angioplasty, intra-arterial papaverine, and intra-arterial nicardipine. Neurosurg Clin N Am 16(3):501–516; vi
14. Kim JH, Park IS, Park KB, Kang DH, Hwang SH (2009) Intraarterial nimodipine infusion to treat symptomatic cerebral vasospasm after aneurysmal subarachnoid hemorrhage. J Korean Neurosurg Soc 46(3):239–244, Epub 2009 Sep 30
15. Komotar RJ, Zacharia BE, Otten ML, Mocco J, Lavine SD (2008) Controversies in the endovascular management of cerebral vasospasm after intracranial aneurysm rupture and future directions for therapeutic approaches. Neurosurgery 62(4):897–905; discussion 905–907
16. Liu JK, Couldwell WT (2005) Intra-arterial papaverine infusions for the treatment of cerebral vasospasm induced by aneurysmal subarachnoid hemorrhage. Neurocrit Care 2(2):124–132
17. Liu JK, Tenner MS, Gottfried ON, Stevens EA, Rosenow JM, Madan N, MacDonald JD, Kestle JR, Couldwell WT (2004) Efficacy of multiple intraarterial papaverine infusions for improvement in cerebral circulation time in patients with recurrent cerebral vasospasm. J Neurosurg 100(3):414–421
18. Mayberg MR (1998) Cerebral vasospasm. Neurosurg Clin N Am 9(3):615–627
19. Mazumdar A, Rivet DJ, Derdeyn CP, Cross DT 3rd, Moran CJ (2006) Effect of intraarterial verapamil on the diameter of vasospastic intracranial arteries in patients with cerebral vasospasm. Neurosurg Focus 21(3):E15
20. McGirt MJ, Garces Ambrossi GL, Huang J, Tamargo RJ (2009) Simvastatin for the prevention of symptomatic cerebral vasospasm following aneurysmal subarachnoid hemorrhage: a single-institution prospective cohort study. J Neurosurg 110(5):968–974
21. Mindea SA, Yang BP, Bendok BR, Miller JW, Batjer HH (2006) Endovascular treatment strategies for cerebral vasospasm. Neurosurg Focus 21(3):E13
22. Newell DW, Eskridge JM, Mayberg MR, Grady MS, Winn HR (1989) Angioplasty for the treatment of symptomatic vasospasm following subarachnoid hemorrhage. J Neurosurg 71(5 Pt 1):654–660
23. Nogueira RG, Lev MH, Roccatagliata L, Hirsch JA, Gonzalez RG, Ogilvy CS, Halpern EF, Rordorf GA, Rabinov JD, Pryor JC (2009) Intra-arterial nicardipine infusion improves CT perfusion-measured cerebral blood flow in patients with subarachnoid hemorrhage-induced vasospasm. AJNR Am J Neuroradiol 30(1):160–164
24. Sayama CM, Liu JK, Couldwell WT (2006) Update on endovascular therapies for cerebral vasospasm induced by aneurysmal subarachnoid hemorrhage. Neurosurg Focus 21(3):E12
25. Sillberg VA, Wells GA, Perry JJ (2008) Do statins improve outcomes and reduce the incidence of vasospasm after aneurysmal subarachnoid hemorrhage: a meta-analysis. Stroke 39(9): 2622–2626
26. Simeone FA, Trepper P (1972) Cerebral vasospasm with infarction. Stroke 3(4):449–455
27. van den Bergh WM (2009) Magnesium in subarachnoid haemorrhage: proven beneficial? Neurocrit Care 11(2):190–198
28. van den Bergh WM, Dijkhuizen RM, Rinkel GJ (2004) Potentials of magnesium treatment in subarachnoid haemorrhage. Magnes Res 17(4):301–313
29. Vergouwen MD, de Haan RJ, Vermeulen M, Roos YB (2010) Effect of statin treatment on vasospasm, delayed cerebral ischemia, and functional outcome in patients with aneurysmal subarachnoid hemorrhage: a systematic review and meta-analysis update. Stroke 41(1):e47–e52
30. Veyna RS, Seyfried D, Burke DG, Zimmerman C, Mlynarek M, Nichols V, Marrocco A, Thomas AJ, Mitsias PD, Malik GM (2002) Magnesium sulfate therapy after aneurysmal subarachnoid hemorrhage. J Neurosurg 96(3):510–514
31. Weir B, Erasmo R, Miller J, McIntyre J, Secord D, Mielke B (1970) Vasospasm in response to repeated subarachnoid hemorrhages in the monkey. J Neurosurg 33(4):395–406
32. Wong GK, Chan MT, Boet R, Poon WS, Gin T (2006) Intravenous magnesium sulfate after aneurysmal subarachnoid hemorrhage: a prospective randomized pilot study. J Neurosurg Anesthesiol 18(2):142–148
33. Wong GK, Chan MT, Poon WS, Boet R, Gin T (2006) Magnesium therapy within 48 hours of an aneurysmal subarachnoid hemorrhage: neuro-panacea. Neurol Res 28(4):431–435

Neck Clipping of Paraclinoid Small Aneurysms

Kenji Kanamaru, Tomohiro Araki, Kazuhide Hamada, Hideki Kanamaru, and Hidenori Suzuki

Abstract Paraclinoid small aneurysms with a diameter less than 5 mm may be difficult to handle intraoperatively. We have encountered 9 such aneurysms among 375 cases. The most frequent location was the ophthalmic segment ($n=6$) followed by the anterior wall ($n=3$) of the internal carotid artery (ICA). The endovascular procedure was not suitable for this particular lesion because of the difficulty in deploying the coil across such small aneurysms. One patient with an ophthalmic segment aneurysm underwent endovascular treatment first; however, the procedure was aborted because of mechanical vasospasm. Finally the patient underwent craniotomy, and the aneurysm was successfully clipped. Two patients with anterior wall aneurysms presented with subarachnoid hemorrhage, and the blood blister-like aneurysms were clipped without sacrifice of the ICA. Five patients with unruptured aneurysms of the ophthalmic segment and one such case of the anterior wall of ICA were all clipped uneventfully. The operative procedure for these small aneurysms is deemed straightforward: (1) high attention should be paid to avoid premature rupture; (2) both the internal carotid artery and optic nerve are mobilized and the anterior clinoid process and falciform ligament are removed, then the aneurysmal neck is created; (3) the neck of the aneurysm is created by pushing the wall of the ICA slightly away during clip application; this is called the "nip on method." Although neck clipping of small aneurysms can be difficult, no efforts should be spared to accomplish direct neck clipping.

Keywords Small aneurysm · Paraclinoid segment of internal carotid artery · Blood blister-like aneurysm · Direct neck clipping

K. Kanamaru (✉), T. Araki, K. Hamada, and H. Kanamaru
Department of Neurosurgery, Suzuka Kaisei Hospital, Suzuka, Japan
e-mail: kanamaru@h6.dion.ne.jp

H. Suzuki
Department of Neurosurgery, Mie University School of Medicine, Tsu, Japan

Introduction

The International Study of Unruptured Intracranial Aneurysms (ISUIA) reported that in the absence of a history of previous rupture, the risk of rupture for small (<7 mm) anterior circulation aneurysms is low, only 0.1% per year [8]. However, many experienced neurosurgeons and endovascular therapists report that in practice, most ruptured aneurysms encountered are small [2, 7]. According to other reports, the extent of SAH after rupture of small aneurysms is often greater than after rupture of larger aneurysms [6, 7]. Despite the advent of sophisticated endovascular materials, embolization of very small aneurysms is associated with relatively high rates of intraprocedural rupture, especially intraoperative rupture [4]. From the surgical point of view, blood blister-like aneurysms arising from the anterior wall of the internal carotid artery (ICA) can be devastating once they rupture [3]. In the present study we demonstrate nine cases of small aneurysms in the paraclinoid segment of the ICA, all of which were successfully clipped.

Materials and Methods

Patients included five women and four men, 41–66 years of age (mean 56 years) (Table 1). Case 3 was referred from another institute because of failure of an endovascular procedure. Key points of the surgical procedures were as follows: (1) frontotemporal craniotomy with removal of the sphenoid ridge; (2) opening of the sylvian fissure as much as possible; (3) removal of the anterior clinoid process and falciform ligament to create sufficient space for clip application; (4) dural adherence to the aneurysm left intact for the protection of the thin aneurysm dome; (5) touching the dome of the aneurysm before neck clipping should be avoided; (6) an angled clip is suitable for anterior wall aneurysms and a straight one for ophthalmic artery aneurysms; (7) additional wrapping and coating may be necessary for anterior wall aneurysms if the parent artery is affected entirely.

DOI: 10.1007/978-3-7091-0661-7_17,

Table 1 Summary of clinical characteristics and clinical outcomes

Case no.	Age (years)	Sex	Initial symptoms	An. location	GOS score
1	46	F	SAH	Rt IC-Ant, IC-PC	5
2	54	F	SAH	Rt IC-Ant, ACA,MCA	5
3	56	M	No	Rt IC-OphA	5
4	65	F	No	Rt IC-OphA	5
5	58	M	No	Lt IC-Ant	5
6	52	M	No	Lt IC-OphA	5
7	66	F	No	Rt IC-OphA	5
8	41	M	No	Lt IC-OphA	5
9	64	F	No	Rt IC-OphA	5

SAH subarachnoid hemorrhage, *IC-Ant* anterior wall of internal carotid artery, *ICPC* internal carotid artery-posterior communicating artery, *ACA* anterior cerebral artery, *MCA* middle cerebral artery, *IC-OphA* internal carotid artery-ophthalmic artery, *An* aneurysm

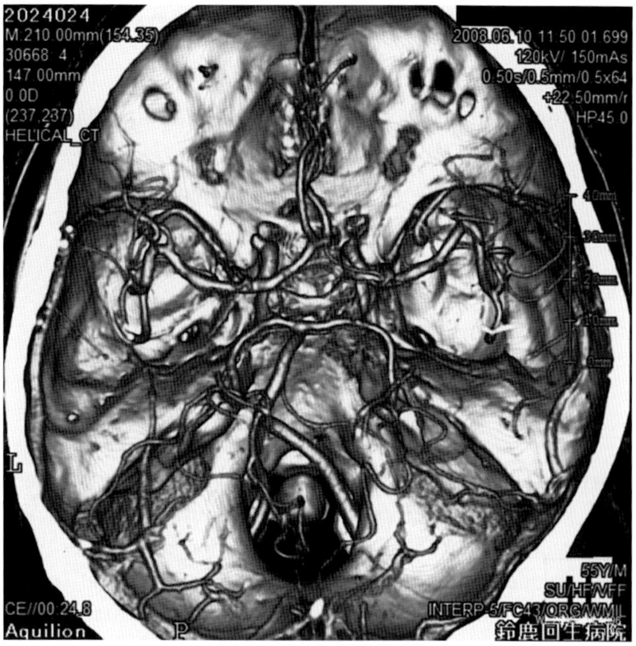

Fig. 1 Preoperative contrast-enhanced CT scans showing left ICA aneurysm arising from the anterior wall

Results

All patients underwent direct surgery of the aneurysm, and neck clipping was successfully performed. There were no perioperative complications. The Glasgow outcome scale score after 3 months demonstrated excellent results in all patients (Table 1).

Illustrative Case

This 58-year-old man with the diagnosis of cerebral aneurysm was referred to us for treatment. The patient had a brain examination using 0.5-T MRI at the Department of Health Services at our institute. Three-dimensional CT scans and angiograms revealed an unruptured small aneurysm with a diameter of 3.4 mm arising from the anterior wall of the left ICA (Fig. 1). Complete obliteration of the aneurysm was achieved uneventfully via craniotomy (Fig. 2). No aneurysm recurrence has been noted for 2 years.

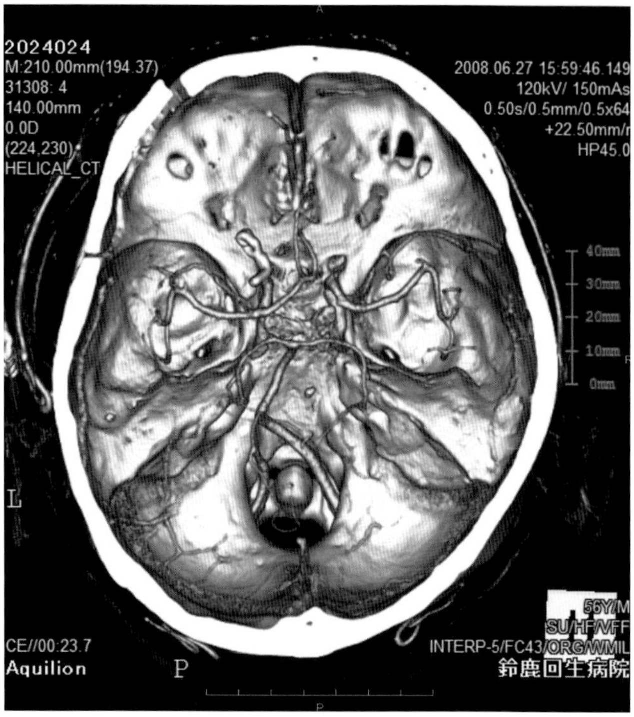

Fig. 2 Postoperative contrast-enhanced CT scans showing complete neck clipping of anterior wall aneurysm of ICA

Discussion

Aneurysms arising from the ICA between the site of its exit from the roof of the cavernous sinus and the origin of the posterior communicating artery have been collectively termed paraclinoid aneurysms [3]. Endovascular therapy for superiorly projecting paraclinoid aneurysms is associated with lower rates of complete obliteration than direct surgery and with rates of cerebral embolic events comparable to those of endovascular treatment in the other groups [3]. Furthermore, endovascular treatment for group II (true ophthalmic artery) aneurysms entails additional risks of retinal embolism [3]. Therefore, direct surgery is recommended for the treatment of paraclinoid aneurysms projecting superiorly [3]. For other groups, especially for group III (carotid cave) aneurysms, endovascular treatment is the acceptable first option of therapy [3]. We agree with the treatment protocol for paraclinoid aneurysms mentioned above. No doubt, overall morbidity and mortality for treatment of an intracranial aneurysm are much lower when treated before rupturing. The risk of surgery must be less than the risk of conservative management (observation) to be recommended. The optimal management of unruptured (incidental) aneurysms continues to be the center of controversy. Recent studies demonstrated that endovascular coil embolization of very small aneurysms <3 mm is associated with relatively high rates of intraprocedural rupture, especially intraoperative rupture [4]. Aneurysms arising from the anterior wall of the ICA, so-called blood blister-like aneurysms (BBA), are rare, reportedly 0.3–1% of intracranial aneurysms or 0.9–6.5% of aneurysms of the ICA [1]. Direct clipping often causes laceration of the lesion, whereas complete wrapping or clipping is effective, but may fail to prevent growth of the aneurysm [1]. A recent study demonstrated that the stent-within-a-stent and covered-stent techniques effectively prevented bleeding and re-growth of the BBA without sacrifice of the ICA [5]. However, the long-term outcome after such a double-stent technique remains unclear. In this study, we successfully treated three cases of BBA. Despite the small number of patients, BBAs could be neck clipped without sacrifice of the ICA. A special technique should be used to clip the BBA, i.e., create a concrete closure line of neck clipping by pushing the wall of ICA slightly away with clip blades. We call this method the "nip on method." In conclusion, neck clipping of small aneurysms can be difficult; however, no efforts should be spared to accomplish direct neck clipping.

Conflict of interest statement We declare that we have no conflict of interest.

References

1. Abe M, Tabuchi K, Yokoyama H, Uchino A (1998) Blood blister-like aneurysms of the internal carotid artery. J Neurosurg 89:419–424
2. Forget TR, Benitez R, Veznedaroglu E, Sharan A, Mitchell W, Silva M, Rosenwasser RH (2001) A review of size and location of ruptured intracranial aneurysms. Neurosurgery 49:1322–1326
3. Iihara K, Murao K, Sakai N, Shindo A, Sakai H, Higashi T, Kogure S, Takahashi JC, Hayashi K, Ishibashi T, Nagata I (2003) Unruptured paraclinoid aneurysms: a management strategy. J Neurosurg 99:241–247
4. Ioannidis I, Lalloo S, Corkill R, Kuker W, Byrne J (2010) Endovascular treatment of very small intracranial aneurysms. J Neurosurg 112:551–556
5. Lee BH, Kim BM, Park MD, Park SI, Chung EC, Suh SH, Choi CS, Won YS, Yu K (2009) Reconstructive endovascular treatment of ruptured blood blister-like aneurysms of the internal carotid artery. J Neurosurg 110:431–436
6. Roos EJ, Rinkel GJ, Velthuis BK, Algra A (2000) The relation between aneurysm size and outcome in patients with subarachnoid hemorrhage. Neurology 54:2334–2336
7. Russell SM, Lin K, Hahn SA, Jafar JJ (2003) Smaller cerebral aneurysms producing more extensive subarachnoid hemorrhage following rupture: a radiological investigation and discussion of theoretical determinants. J Neurosurg 99:248–253
8. Wiebers DO, Whisnant JP, Huston J III, Meissner I, Brown RD Jr, Piepgras DG et al (2003) Unruptured intracranial aneurysms: natural history, clinical outcome, and risks of surgical and endovascular treatment. Lancet 362:103–110

Deferoxamine Reduces Early Brain Injury Following Subarachnoid Hemorrhage

Jin-Yul Lee, Richard F. Keep, Ya Hua, Ralf-Ingo Ernestus, and Guohua Xi

Abstract The effect of subarachnoid hemoglobin on neuroglial cells contributing to early brain injury is unclear. Several intracerebral hemorrhage studies indicated that pathological iron deposition in the brain contributes to secondary brain injury. Therefore, the purpose of this study was to investigate the relationship between iron and neuroglial cell changes following SAH, and examine the effect of deferoxamine (DFX). SAH was induced in male Sprague-Dawley rats ($n=56$) using an endovascular perforation technique. Animals were treated with DFX (100 mg/kg) or vehicle for 3 days. Rats were sacrificed at 6 h, days 1 and 3 to determine non-heme iron and heme oxygenase (HO)-1 expression using Western blot and immunohistochemistry analysis. To assess neuronal cell death, Fluoro-Jade- and terminal deoxynucleotidyl transferase-mediated dUTP nick end-labeling (TUNEL) stainings were performed. Marked HO-1 upregulation at day 3 ($P<0.01$) was accompanied by elevated non-heme iron ($P<0.01$) and ferritin levels ($P<0.01$). DFX treatment reduced brain non-heme iron concentration, ferritin expression and neuronal cell death at day 3 ($P<0.01$) following SAH. These results suggest that excessive hemoglobin and iron overload play an important role in early brain injury following SAH. Acute treatment with DFX significantly ameliorates neuronal cell death and may be a potential therapeutic agent for SAH.

Keywords Deferoxamine · Hemoglobin · Iron · Neuronal death · Subarachnoid hemorrhage

J.-Y. Lee (✉)
Department of Neurosurgery, University of Würzburg, Josef-Schneider-Str. 11, 97080 Würzburg, Germany
e-mail: jinannarbor@gmail.com

R.F. Keep, Y. Hua, and G. Xi
Department of Neurosurgery, University of Michigan, Ann Arbor, MI, USA

R.-I. Ernestus
Department of Neurosurgery, University of Würzburg, Würzburg, Germany

Introduction

Aneurysmal subarachnoid hemorrhage (SAH) is a severe disease causing high mortality, especially within the first few days [1]. Although the combination of increased intracranial pressure and decreased cerebral blood flow resulting in global cerebral ischemia plays an important role, the underlying injury mechanisms during this early period remain poorly understood. Following SAH, the brain is exposed to a great amount of hemoglobin as erythrocytes lyse, especially at the basal surface of the brain [6]. Blood released into the subarachnoid space clots almost immediately, and clot lysis starts early after SAH [8]. Heme is degraded in the brain by heme-oxygenase (HO) into carbon monoxide and biliverdin with the release of catalytically active iron, which may participate in the formation of the highly reactive hydroxyl radical via Fenton reaction [12]. DFX has been used in clinical practice for more than 30 years in iron-overloaded patients with acute iron intoxication or overload due to transfusion-dependent anemia. It is a hydrophilic chelator that has a high affinity for ferric iron, forming a stable complex that prevents the iron from entering into further chemical reactions [9]. This study focuses on the role of subarachnoid hemoglobin and iron in brain injury during the acute phase of SAH and examines the effect of DFX on SAH-induced injury.

Materials and Methods

Fifty-six male Sprague-Dawley rats weighing 275–325 g were used. General anesthesia was induced with 5% isoflurane (Aerrane; Baxter Healthcare Corp., Deerfield, IL). After intubation and initiation of mechanical ventilation, isoflurane was titrated between 2.25% and 2.75% to maintain a mean arterial pressure between 80 and 120 mmHg.

T. Tsukahara et al. (eds.), *Trends in Neurovascular Surgery*, Acta Neurochirurgica Supplementum, Vol. 112,
DOI: 10.1007/978-3-7091-0661-7_18,

SAH Induction

In supine position and after a left paramedian incision of the ventral neck, the left external carotid artery was identified under a surgical microscope, and transected distally. A 3-0 nylon monofilament suture with a rounded tip to prevent endothelial injury was inserted, advanced distally into the intracranial internal carotid artery and carefully perforated under intracranial pressure (ICP) monitoring. Sham-operated control rats underwent an identical procedure without vessel perforation. The suture was withdrawn 5 min after insertion. DFX (100 mg/kg) was administered i.p. 2 h and 6 h post-hemorrhage followed by every 12 h for 3 days.

Grading of SAH

The basal brain including brainstem was divided into six segments (anterior and posterior circle of Willis on both sides and left and right brainstem). Each segment was assigned a grade from 0 to 3 depending on the amount of subarachnoid blood clot as follows; grade 0: no subarachnoid blood; grade 1: minimal subarachnoid blood; grade 2: moderate blood clot with recognizable arteries; grade 3: blood clot covering the cerebral arteries. The blood distribution in the ventrolateral brainstem was also considered grade 2 and 3 depending on the amount of blood.

Non-heme Brain Tissue Iron Determination

Following extensive perfusion with 0.1 mol/l phosphate-buffered saline (pH 7.4) and brain removal, the remaining subarachnoid blood was carefully removed from the basal surface of the brain. A coronal slice of brain ~4 mm thick around the optic chiasm was cut. The ipsilateral frontobasal cortex was separated and weighed. After homogenization of the brain samples, 1 ml of 8.5 mol/l HCl added and hydrolyzed at 90°C for 60 min. Following cooling, 2 ml of 20% trichloroacetic acid was added to precipitate proteins, and the supernatant collected after centrifugation. The supernatant was then run through an acid-washed filter and the precipitate washed with 1 ml of 4.25 mol/l HCl plus 20% trichloroacetic acid (1:1). The supernatant was collected and 4 ml of 1 mol/l sodium citrate added. The pH was adjusted to 3.1 and the final volume adjusted to 25 ml. The total non-heme iron concentration was assayed by a spectrophotometer with ferrozine as color reagent.

Western Blot Analysis

After removal of the brain, a 3-mm-thick ipsilateral frontobasal cortex sample was separated at the level of the optic chiasm. Primary antibodies were: polyclonal rabbit anti-horse spleen ferritin (Sigma, 1:250 dilution) or polyclonal rabbit anti-rat HO-1 (StressGen; 1:2,500 dilution). Antigen-antibody complexes were visualized with the ECL chemiluminescence system (Amersham) and exposed to Kodak X-OMAT film. Relative band densities were analyzed with an NIH Image program (version 1.61).

Immunohistochemistry

Rats underwent intracardiac perfusion with 4% paraformaldehyde in 0.1 mol/l phosphate-buffered saline (pH 7.4). Brains were removed and kept in 4% paraformaldehyde for 12 h, then immersed in 25% sucrose for 3 days at 4°C. Brains were then placed in embedding compound and sectioned (18 μm) on a cryostat. Immunohistochemical staining was performed using the avidin-biotin complex technique. Primary antibodies were polyclonal rabbit anti-rat HO-1 (StressGen; 1:400 dilution) and rabbit anti-human ferritin (DAKO; 1:100 dilution). Normal rabbit IgG (Vector Laboratories, Burlingame, CA) was used as a negative control. To detect DNA fragmentation, sections were processed for terminal deoxynucleotidyl transferase-mediated dUTP nick end-labeling (TUNEL) using an in situ cell death detection kit (Intergen). Cell counting was conducted in the basal cerebral cortex on 40× microscopic images using a CK-2 Olympus microscope. Positive cells were counted in three separate fields in three different slices cut at the level of the optic chiasm.

Statistical Analysis

Values are presented as mean ± SD. Statistical comparisons between groups were performed using one-way analysis of variance (ANOVA) followed by either a Dunnett's or a Tukey's post-hoc test, the former for comparisons to a single control group, the latter to compare across multiple groups. Mortality was compared with a chi-squared test. A probability of $P<0.05$ was considered statistically significant.

Results

SAH Extent and Mortality Rate

No sham-operated control animals died. All animals in both groups had extensive SAH. This was particularly pronounced on the ipsilateral side, around the circle of Willis and along the ventral brainstem. At 24 h post hemorrhage, the SAH score was 14 ± 3 and 13 ± 2 out of a possible 18 in the SAH groups without and with DFX treatment, respectively. DFX treatment decreased the mortality rate to 21% (32% in the SAH group without DFX).

Increased HO-1 Expression After SAH

SAH was accompanied by significant upregulation in hemoxygenase (HO)-1 expression (13,529 ± 1,802 pixels, $P<0.01$) compared with sham-operated control (7,634 ± 2,409). HO-1 positive cells were detected in the cortical area of the basal brain, and the immunoreactivity was predominantly localized to microglia. Treatment with DFX greatly reduced the induction of HO-1 by SAH (8,677 ± 3,621, $P<0.05$, Fig. 1).

Non-heme Iron Concentration and Ferritin Levels in the Brain Tissue

Brain non-heme iron levels increased progressively in vehicle-treated SAH rats, reaching a maximum 3 days after SAH (101 ± 16 vs. 43 ± 10 μg/g brain tissue in the sham-operated control group, $P<0.01$). Accordingly, ferritin levels also increased significantly on day 3 following SAH (6,693 ± 1,596 vs. 1,474 ± 797 pixels in sham-operated controls, $P<0.01$). This increase in non-heme iron and ferritin after SAH was markedly reduced by systemic DFX treatment (64 ± 17 μg/g brain tissue at day 3, $P<0.05$, and 3,074 ± 557, $P<0.01$, respectively). Double labeling

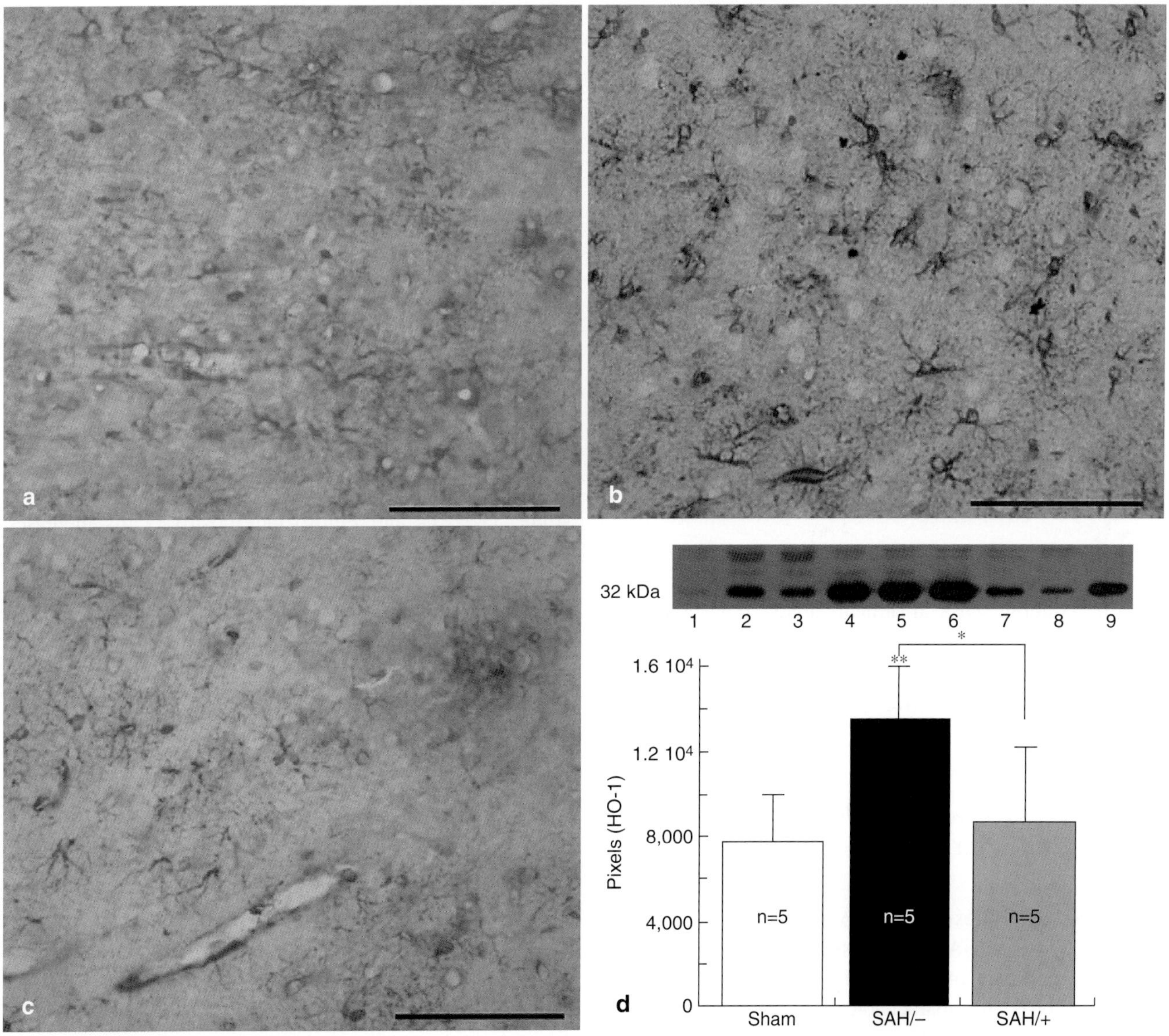

Fig. 1 HO-1 immunoreactivities in the ipsilateral frontal cortex 24 h following sham-operation (**a**) or SAH without (**b**) and with DFX treatment (**c**). Scale bar = 100 μm. (**d**) Western blot analysis showing significant increase in cortical HO-1 expression 24 h after SAH induction (SAH/–, lanes 4–6) compared to the sham-operated control group (lanes 1–3). SAH rats with DFX treatment (SAH/+, lanes 7–9) exhibited significantly decreased HO-1 expression. Values are mean ± SD. $^{*}P<0.05$ and $^{**}P<0.01$ versus sham

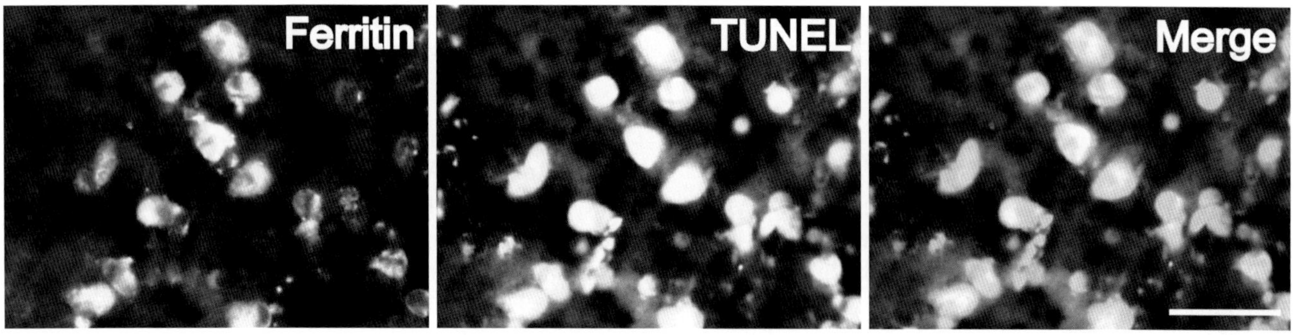

Fig. 2 Double immunofluorescent labeling for ferritin and TUNEL. Ferritin-positive cells exhibit DNA damage, indicating apoptotic cell death. Scale bar = 50 μm

demonstrated that most ferritin-positive cells were either microglial cells or neurons. Furthermore, most TUNEL-positive cells were ferritin-positive and neuron-like (Fig. 2).

Neuronal Cell Death and Oxidative DNA Injury

Fluoro-Jade stains the cell bodies, dendrites and axons of dying neurons. Fluoro-Jade-positive cells were observed in the ipsilateral fronto-basal brain 24 h following SAH (Fig. 3e–i). Correspondingly, numerous TUNEL-positive cells were found in the cortical and subcortical area of the basal brain at day 1 and further increased at day 3 after hemorrhage. DFX treatment caused a significant reduction in Fluoro-Jade- and TUNEL-positive cells, resulting in markedly fewer brain lesions (Fig. 3f, i).

Discussion

SAH induced marked increases in brain non-heme iron and ferritin. Systemic DFX treatment largely prevented those changes and reduced SAH-induced cell damage. Together, these results suggest that iron may be a target for reducing acute brain injury after SAH.

HO-1 Expression, Non-heme Iron and Ferritin After SAH

In this study, HO-1 expression rapidly increased in the basal brain at day 1 after SAH and peaked at day 3. This response might be the result of intraparenchymal hemoglobin overload after lysis of subarachnoid erythrocytes. Heme is a potent inducer of HO-1 [12]. However, HO-1 can be induced by a wide variety of the factors including hydroxyl radicals [11]. Our finding that DFX blunted SAH-induced HO-1 upregulation suggests that iron-mediated free radical production contributes to the upregulation or that DFX interferes with the induction of HO-1 by heme.

Increased Cell Death

Iron is an essential element needed for neuronal development, myelination and synthesis of neurotransmitters [2]. Abnormally high levels of iron, however, can lead to significant oxidative damage via free radical production within the brain [2]. Several of our prior studies have demonstrated that iron deposition after ICH causes oxidative injury resulting in brain edema, neuronal cell death and delayed brain atrophy [4, 10]. The degree of brain lesion correlates directly with regional iron concentration [5]. TUNEL and Fluoro-Jade stainings are sensitive markers of DNA damage and neuronal cell death [3]. In the current study, TUNEL- and Fluoro-Jade-positive cells increased progressively on days 1 and 3 after SAH induction, suggesting that DNA damage and cell death may be an important injury mechanism after SAH. Such DNA damage and neuronal cell death were markedly reduced by DFX treatment, indicating a potential role of iron in that damage. Co-localization studies of TUNEL with ferritin indicated that the majority of dying cells were ferritin-positive and neuron-like.

Deferoxamine

DFX is rapidly absorbed and can easily penetrate the blood barrier, leading to accumulation in the brain tissue at a significant concentration following systemic administration [9]. Several mechanisms underlying neuroprotective functions of DFX have been proposed. These include chelation of the

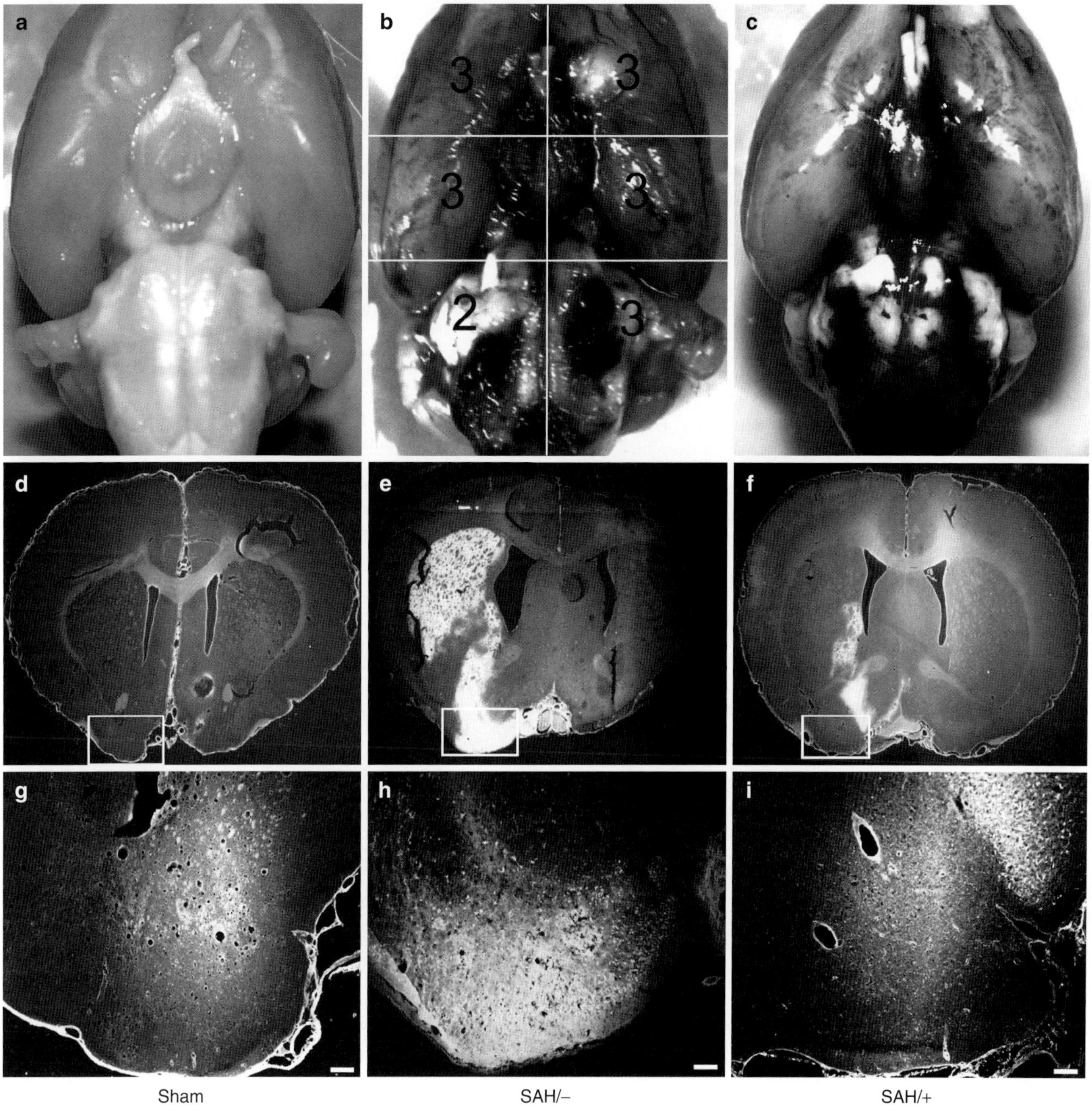

Fig. 3 Macroscopic and histologic pictures with corresponding Fluoro-Jade staining at the level of optic chiasm 24 h following sham operation (**a**, **d**, **g**) or SAH induction without (**b**, **e**, **h**) and with DFX treatment (**c**, **f**, **i**). For the assessment of SAH extent, the basal brain surface was divided into six segments and each segment rated for hemorrhage (**b**). SAH caused an extensive lesion in the ipsilateral frontobasal brain, adjacent to the subarachnoid blood clot (**e**, **h**). Despite similar SAH extent and distribution, the treatment with DFX resulted in markedly less cerebral lesion (**f**, **i**). Scale bar = 100 μm

unbound labile iron responsible for catalyzing the production of reactive oxygen species and the subsequent modulation of gene expression, including the HIF-1α, and blocking neurotoxic effects of hemoglobin through inhibition of glutamate-mediated excitotoxicity [7, 9].

In this study, DFX markedly reduced brain non-heme iron and, probably as a consequence, also lowered the expression of ferritin. Moreover, TUNEL- and Fluoro-Jade-labeled cell death was reduced. These findings suggest that DFX effectively diminished hydroxyl radical formation and oxidative stress by sequestering redox-active iron.

Acknowledgement This study was supported by the Else Kröner-Fresenius-Stiftung, Bad Homburg, Germany, and Stiftung Neurochirurgische Forschung der Deutschen Gesellschaft für Neurochirurgie, Germany.

Conflict of interest statement We declare that we have no conflict of interest.

References

1. Broderick JP, Brott TG, Duldner JE, Tomsick T, Leach A (1994) Initial and recurrent bleeding are the major causes of death following subarachnoid hemorrhage. Stroke 25:1342–1347
2. Carbonell T, Rama R (2007) Iron, oxidative stress and early neurological deterioration in ischemic stroke. Curr Med Chem 14:857–874
3. Chen K, Jin K, Chen M, Pei W, Kawaguchi K, Greenberg DA, Simon RP (1997) Early detection of DNA strand breaks in the brain after transient focal ischemia: implications for the role of DNA damage in apoptosis and neuronal cell death. J Neurochem 69:232–245
4. Hua Y, Nakamura T, Keep RF, Wu J, Schallert T, Hoff JT, Xi G (2006) Long-term effects of experimental intracerebral hemorrhage: the role of iron. J Neurosurg 104:305–312
5. Koeppen AH, Dickson AC, McEvoy JA (1995) The cellular reactions to experimental intracerebral hemorrhage. J Neurol Sci 134: 102–112
6. Lee J-Y, Sagher O, Keep R, Hua Y, Xi G (2009) Comparison of experimental rat models of early brain injury after subarachnoid hemorrhage. Neurosurgery 65:331–343
7. Nakamura T, Keep RF, Hua Y, Schallert T, Hoff JT, Xi G (2004) Deferoxamine-induced attenuation of brain edema and neurological deficits in a rat model of intracerebral hemorrhage. J Neurosurg 100:672–678
8. Nina P, Schisano G, Chiappetta F, Luisa Papa M, Maddaloni E, Brunori A, Capasso F, Corpetti MG, Demurtas F (2001) A study of blood coagulation and fibrinolytic system in spontaneous subarachnoid hemorrhage. Correlation with Hunt-Hess grade and outcome. Surg Neurol 55:197–203
9. Palmer C, Roberts RL, Bero C (1994) Deferoxamine posttreatment reduces ischemic brain injury in neonatal rats. Stroke 25: 1039–1045
10. Song S, Hua Y, Keep RF, Hoff JT, Xi G (2007) A new hippocampal model for examining intracerebral hemorrhage-related neuronal death. Stroke 38:2861–2863
11. Syapin PJ (2009) Regulation of haeme oxygenase-1 for treatment of neuroinflammation and brain disorders. Br J Pharmacol 155:623–640
12. Wagner KR, Sharp FR, Ardizzone TD, Lu A, Clark JF (2003) Heme and iron metabolism: role in cerebral hemorrhage. J Cereb Blood Flow Metab 23:629–652

Does Magnetic Resonance Imaging Produce Further Benefit for Detecting a Bleeding Source in Subarachnoid Hemorrhage of Unknown Origin?

Homajoun Maslehaty, Athanassios K. Petridis, Harald Barth, Alexandros Doukas, and Hubertus Maximilian Mehdorn

Abstract *Background:* Spontaneous subarachnoid hemorrhage (SAH) without evidence of a bleeding source on the first digital subtraction angiogram (DSA) – also called SAH of unknown origin – is observed in up to 27% of all cases. Depending on the bleeding pattern on CT scanning, SAH can be differentiated into perimesencephalic (PM-SAH) and non-perimesencephalic SAH (NON-PM-SAH). The aim of our study was to investigate the effectiveness of magnetic resonance imaging (MRI) for detecting a bleeding source in SAH of unknown origin.

Methods: We retrospectively reviewed 1,226 patients with spontaneous SAH between January 1991 and December 2008 in our department. DSA was performed in 1,068 patients, with negative results in 179 patients.

Results: Forty-seven patients were categorized as having PM-SAH and 132 patients as having NON-PM-SAH. MRI of the brain and the craniocervical region was performed within 72 h after diagnosis of SAH and demonstrated no bleeding sources in any of the PM-SAH and NON-PM-SAH patients (100% negative).

Conclusions: In our experience MRI did not produce any additional benefit for detecting a bleeding source after SAH with a negative angiogram. The costs of this examination exceeded the clinical value. Despite our results MRI should be discussed on a case-by-case basis because rare bleeding sources are periodically diagnosed in cases of NON-PM-SAH.

Keywords Perimesencephalic subarachnoid hemorrhage · Subarachnoid hemorrhage of unknown origin · Non-aneurysmal subarachnoid hemorrhage · Diagnostic magnetic resonance imaging

Introduction

Spontaneous subarachnoid hemorrhage (SAH) is most often associated with ruptured intracranial aneurysms (70–80%), and less frequently with arteriovenous malformations (4%). If a bleeding source is not identified on the initial cerebral digital subtraction angiogram (DSA), it is called SAH of unknown origin [2, 3, 5, 10–12].

Depending on the bleeding pattern on CT, SAH of unknown origin can be subdivided into perimesencephalic (PM-SAH) and non-perimesencephalic SAH (NON-PM-SAH). PM-SAH is defined as blood accumulation in the perimesencephalic, interpeduncular and prepontine cisterns, without involvement of brain parenchyma, the ventricular system or the sylvian fissure. If the mentioned areas are involved, SAH can be categorized as NON-PM-SAH [2, 4, 12, 14, 16].

The aim of our study was to investigate the effectiveness of magnetic resonance imaging (MRI) for detecting a bleeding source in SAH of unknown origin.

Material and Methods

We retrospectively reviewed all patients with spontaneous SAH in our department between January 1991 and December 2008 ($n = 1,226$) through an analysis of our database. Patients with traumatic SAH and unclear history were excluded from the study. Diagnosis was made by CT scanning, and blood accumulation was scored using the Fisher classification. Four-vessel DSA including additional catheterization of both external carotid arteries was performed in 1,068 patients.

H. Maslehaty (✉)
Department of Neurosurgery, University Hospitals Schleswig-Holstein, Campus Kiel, Arnold-Heller-Strasse 3, 24105 Kiel, Germany
e-mail: h.maslehaty@gmx.de

A.K. Petridis, H. Barth, A. Doukas, and H.M. Mehdorn
Department of Neurosurgery, University Hospitals Schleswig-Holstein, Campus Kiel, Kiel, Germany

T. Tsukahara et al. (eds.), *Trends in Neurovascular Surgery*, Acta Neurochirurgica Supplementum, Vol. 112,
DOI: 10.1007/978-3-7091-0661-7_19, © Springer-Verlag/Wien 2011

The remaining 158 patients were not examined with DSA because of poor clinical condition (Hunt and Hess 5), rapid death or immediate neurosurgical treatment.

According to the previously mentioned radiological features, patients with initially negative angiograms were divided into two groups. Group 1 included patients with PM-SAH (47 patients) and CT scanning during the first 24 h after occurrence of clinical symptoms. Group 2 included the patients with NON-PM-SAH (132 patients).

All patients underwent standard monitoring and received standard therapy for aneurysmal SAH in the intensive care unit. Clinical condition at the time of presentation was scored using the Hunt and Hess classification. Patients of group 1 and 2 underwent MRI [Phillips® 3-T MRI with T1-weighted spin echo, T2-weighted turbo spin echo, T2-weighted steady-state free precession (FFE), FLAIR, time-of-flight MR angiography and venous bold sequences] of the brain and craniocervical region during the initial 72 h after SAH was diagnosed.

Results

Overall, we analyzed data from 1,226 patients with spontaneous SAH. The results are displayed in Fig. 1. One thousand sixty-eight (87.1%) patients underwent DSA, with negative results in 179 patients (16.7%). Forty-seven patients were categorized as having PM-SAH (group 1, 26.3%) and 132 patients as having NON-PM-SAH (group 2, 73.7%). MRI of the brain and the craniocervical region detected no bleeding sources in groups 1 and 2 (100% negative).

Discussion

Spontaneous SAH is usually caused by ruptured vascular malformations. However, according to several studies a bleeding source is not identified on the first DSA in up to 27% of cases. The reason could be initial local vasospasm or occlusion of the ruptured aneurysm due to blood clots [7, 9–11]. Regarding the differentiation between PM-SAH and NON-PM-SAH, we consider it important to note the radiological features of CT findings. It is also important to perform the initial CT within 24 h after occurrence of symptoms. CT scanning a few days after initial symptoms can lead to false-positive findings because of variance of bleeding patterns and redistribution of blood in the perimesencephalic space.

PM-SAH itself is sometimes considered to be a benign subtype of aneurysmal SAH. Patients most commonly present with crushing headache and meningism, although severe neurological deficits are not generally observed. Hunt and Hess grade at presentation is predominantly 1–2; higher grades are very rare. The clinical course is usually uneventful, without dreaded complications such as re-bleeding and ischemic neurological deficits following cerebral vasospasm. Long-term follow-up examinations revealed a generally good prognosis of PM-SAH [4, 6, 11], although the bleeding source is unclear. Infrequently, PM-SAH results from cerebral microaneurysms, intracranial artery dissection, pituitary apoplexy, intracranial neoplasms, cerebral cavernous hemangiomas or venous leak [8, 15, 16].

Considering the negative initial DSA, a cranial MRI including the craniocervical region is performed routinely at our department to rule out bleeding sources. In reviewing the literature, we found that detecting a bleeding source by MRI is reported very infrequently and exclusively in patients with a NON-PM-SAH [1, 13, 17, 18].

In our series of 47 patients with PM-SAH and 132 with NON-PM-SAH, MRI had 100% negative findings. Considering our results and the published data, it is justified to challenge the indication for MRI examination in SAH of unknown origin. Based on our series, it can be concluded that MRI examination in patients with PM-SAH and NON-PM-SAH did not produce further benefit for detecting a bleeding source and had no consequence for the administered therapy. The costs of MRI examination clearly exceeded the clinical value.

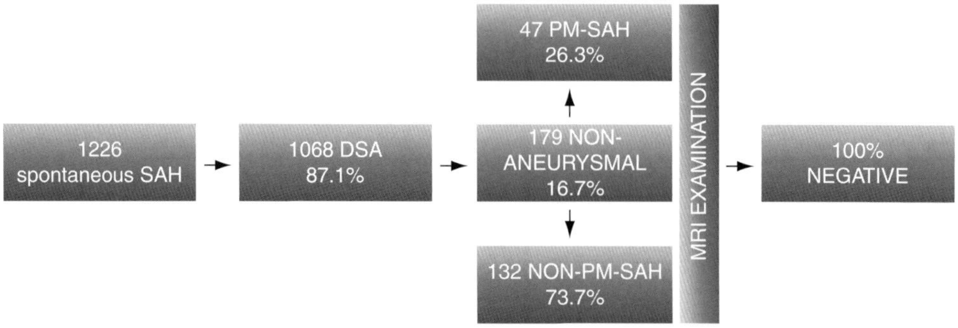

Fig. 1 Flow chart of the diagnostic results

Despite our observations, the option of performing MRI should be discussed for selected patients with atypical forms of NON-PM-SAH to avoid rare constellations such as cervical schwannoma with primarily neck and upper back pain.

The ideal time of examination is still being investigated. It remains to be proven whether MRI should be performed during initial therapy as a later control examination instead of CT scanning, as episodes of re-bleeding have been infrequently reported. Further prospective studies with distinct test conditions are necessary to answer the open questions.

Conclusion

MRI of the brain and craniocervical region added no further benefit for detecting a bleeding source or administering therapy following PM-SAH and NON-PM-SAH in our series (100% negative). The costs of this examination exceeded the clinical value. Despite our results, however, the option of MRI should be discussed on a case-by-case basis, because rare bleeding sources are periodically diagnosed in cases with NON-PM-SAH. Further prospective studies are necessary to verify our observations.

Conflict of interest statement We declare that we have no conflict of interest.

References

1. Andaluz N, Zuccarello M (2008) Yield of further diagnostic work-up of cryptogenic subarachnoid hemorrhage based on bleeding patterns on computed tomographic scans. Neurosurgery 62(5):1040–1046; discussion 1047
2. Barth H, Nabavi A, Stein H, Behnke A, Mehdorn HM (1996) Perimesencephalic subarachnoid hemorrhage - an independent clinical picture of non-aneurysmatic subarachnoid hemorrhage with a benign course. Zentralbl Neurochir 57(2):108–112
3. Berdoz D, Uske A, de Tribolet N (1998) Subarachnoid haemorrhage of unknown cause: clinical, neuroradiological and evolutive aspects. J Clin Neurosci 5(3):274–282
4. Beseoglu K, Pannes S, Steiger HJ, Hänggi D (2010) Long-term outcome and quality of life after nonaneurysmal subarachnoid hemorrhage. Acta Neurochir (Wien) 152(3):409–416
5. Björkesten G, Halonen V (1965) Incidence of intracranial vascular lesions in patients with subarachnoid hemorrhage investigated by four-vessel angiography. J Neurosurg 23(1):29–32
6. Flaherty ML, Haverbusch M, Kissela B, Kleindorfer D, Schneider A, Sekar P, Moomaw CJ, Sauerbeck L, Broderick JP, Woo D (2005) Perimesencephalic subarachnoid hemorrhage: incidence, risk factors, and outcome. J Stroke Cerebrovasc Dis 14(6):267–271
7. Fujii M, Ye T, Masaoka H, Ohta Y, Hayakawa T, Honma M (2006) Analysis of unknown cause subarachnoid hemorrhage with repeated negative angiogram. No To Shinkei 58(6):489–493
8. Germans MR, Pennings FA, Sprengers ME, Vandertop WP (2008) Spinal vascular malformations in non-perimesencephalic subarachnoid hemorrhage. J Neurol 255(12):1910–1915
9. Jung JY, Kim YB, Lee JW, Huh SK, Lee KC (2006) Spontaneous subarachnoid haemorrhage with negative initial angiography: a review of 143 cases. J Clin Neurosci 13(10):1011–1017
10. Lang EW, Khodair A, Barth H, Hempelmann RG, Dorsch NW, Mehdorn HM (2003) Subarachnoid hemorrhage of unknown origin and the basilar artery configuration. J Clin Neurosci 10(1):74–78
11. Mehdorn HM, Dietrich U, Kalff R, Hoffmann B, Rauhut F, Grote W (1992) Subarachnoid hemorrhage of unknown origin. Longterm prognosis. Neurosurg Rev 15(1):27–31
12. Meisenzahl EM, Gottschalk S, Lechner C, Lehmann R (1998) Spontaneous perimesencephalic subarachnoid hemorrhage (PMH). A disease category with good prognosis. Fortschr Neurol Psychiatr 66(9):387–390
13. Rogg JM, Smeaton S, Doberstein C, Goldstein JH, Tung GA (1999) Haas RA (1999) Assessment of the value of MR imaging for examining patients with angiographically negative subarachnoid hemorrhage. AJR Am J Roentgenol 172(1):201–206
14. Schievink WI, Wijdicks EF (1997) Pretruncal subarachnoid hemorrhage: an anatomically correct description of the perimesencephalic subarachnoid hemorrhage. Stroke 28(12):2572
15. Schwartz SH, Solomon RA (1996) Perimesencephalic nonaneurysmal subarachnoid hemorrhage: review of the literature. Neurosurgery 39:433–444
16. Van Gijn J, van Dongen KJ, Vermeulen M, Hijdra A (1995) Perimesencephalic hemorrhage: a nonaneurysmal and benign form of subarachnoid hemorrhage. Neurology 35:493–497
17. Wijdicks EF, Schievink WI, Miller GM (1998) MR imaging in pretruncal nonaneurysmal subarachnoid hemorrhage: is it worthwhile? Stroke 29(12):2514–2516
18. Yamamoto M, Fukushima T, Ikeda K, Nagasaka S, Sakamoto S, Oka K (1993) Intracranial cavernous angioma manifesting as subarachnoid hemorrhage-case report. Neurol Med Chir (Tokyo) 33(10): 706–709

Treatment of Experimental Cerebral Vasospasm by Protein Transduction of Heme Oxygenase 1 (HO-1) Conjugated to a Residue of 11 Arginines

Tomoyuki Ogawa, Daniel Hänggi, and Hans-Jakob Steiger

Abstract *Background*: Many kinds of proteins can be transduced into various cells by conjugation with 10–20 amino acid peptides. A sequence of 11 consecutive arginine groups (11R) is one of the most efficient protein transduction domains (PTD). We used the 32-kDa heat shock protein heme oxygenase-1 (HO-1) as a therapeutic protein for experimental cerebral vasospasm. This protein is an enzyme of the heme-catabolism and cleaves heme to form biliverdin and carbon monoxide (CO). HO-1 has known vascular relaxing properties. We examined the transduction efficacy and antispastic therapeutic effect of 11R fused HO-1 protein in cerebral arteries.

Methods: 11R fused HO-1 protein was expressed purified. An MTT assay was used to evaluate the cytotoxicity of 11R-HO-1. An antispastic effect was investigated in a rat model of experimental subarachnoid hemorrhage by measuring basilar artery diameters 4 h after the injection of 11R-HO-1 into the cisterna.

Findings: Expression and purification of 11R-HO-1 could be successfully effected. Transduction into the basilar artery was also successful. 11R-HO-1 protein has the positive effect of attenuating cerebral vasospasm.

Conclusion: These results suggest that the 11R-HO-1 protein transduction method has a potential to treat cerebral vasospasm.

Keywords Cerebral vasospasm · Protein transduction method · Eleven arginines (11R) · Heme oxygenase 1(HO-1) · Subarachnoid hemorrhage (SAH)

T. Ogawa (✉), D. Hänggi, and H.-J. Steiger
Department of Neurosurgery, Heinrich Heine University, Moorenstraße 5, 40225 Düsseldorf, Germany
e-mail: tomoyuki.ogawa@uni-duesseldorf.de

Introduction

Gene therapy has been widely performed in the research field of cerebrovascular diseases including cerebral vasospasm after SAH. However, previous reports revealed that this method has some drawbacks, for example, viral toxicity, inflammatory response and low transduction efficacy [1, 2, 13, 14, 17]. Alternatively, protein transduction has recently attracted attention as a promising method. By conjugating a protein transduction domain (PTD) to the effector protein, many proteins and peptides can be introduced into virtually any kind of cells [3, 4, 15, 16]. Therefore, we tried to apply this new method to the research field of cerebral vasospasm. Here, we used heme oxygenase 1 (HO-1) [6, 12] as a therapeutic protein and 11 consecutive arginines (11R) [5, 7–11] as a protein transduction domain (PTD) and examined whether protein transduction of 11R-HO-1 in vivo ameliorates cerebral vasoconstriction after SAH.

Materials and Methods

MTT (3-(4, 5-Dimethylthiazol-2-yl)-2, 5-Diphenyltetrazolium Bromide, a Tetrazole) Assay

This assay is based on the cleavage of the yellow tetrazolium salt MTT to purple formazan crystals by metabolic active cells. Cells were incubated with 0.1 μM 11R-HO-1 protein or as a control with enhanced green fluorescent protein (EGFP) conjugated to 11R ($n=7$, each) at 37°C for 24 h. Cells were incubated with the yellow MTT solution. Four hours later, these mediums were solubilized by adding the solubilization solution and incubating the plates at 37°C for 24 h. In this way, the formazan crystals were dissolved, and the resulting color absorption was quantified with a scanning spectrophotometer (ELISA).

T. Tsukahara et al. (eds.), *Trends in Neurovascular Surgery*, Acta Neurochirurgica Supplementum, Vol. 112,
DOI: 10.1007/978-3-7091-0661-7_20, © Springer-Verlag/Wien 2011

Experimental Model of SAH

After examining the protein with MTT assay, a rat double-hemorrhage model of SAH was used to assess whether protein transduction of 11R-HO-1 prevents vasospasm in vivo (Fig. 1). Male Sprague-Dawley rats were randomly assigned to two groups: intracisternal injection of 11R-HO-1 or control (SAH+Saline). On day 0, the animals were anesthetized and allowed to breathe spontaneously, after which 0.2 mL of arterial blood was injected into the cisterna magna over 5 min. The rats were reanesthetized 2 days after the initial injection (day 2) and given a second injection of 0.2 mL of autologous arterial blood. Seven days after the first injection, rats were sacrificed with overdoses of anesthetic agents. Several hours before being euthanized, saline or 11R-HO-1 was injected into the cisterna magna. The animals were fixed by perfusion with 100 mL of PBS at physiological blood pressure. Frozen sections of BA and brainstem were cut 10 μm thick on the cryostat, and BA diameters were measured using a light microscope equipped with a micrometer. Cross sections of BA were obtained for measurement at three points: 200 μm above the union of the vertebral arteries, just below the anterior inferior cerebellar arteries and 200 μm below the BA bifurcation. The average of the three locations was used as the diameter of the BA.

Results

Cytotoxicity of 11R-HO-1

With the cell proliferation assay (MTT assay), the transduction of 11R-HO-1 protein did not inhibit the growth of the cells (Fig. 2).

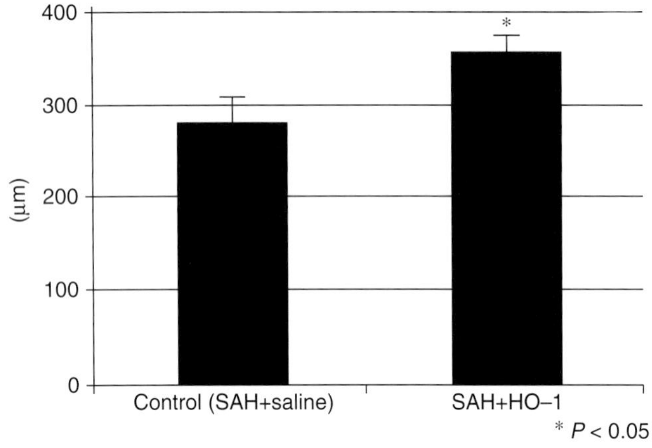

Fig. 1 A rat double-hemorrhage model of SAH was used to assess whether protein transduction of 11R-HO-1 prevents vasospasm in vivo. Basilar artery diameter in the control group (SAH only) was 287.25±19.47 μm and in the 11R-HO-1 injection group 367.21±24.65 μm, $p<0.05$

Therapeutic Effect of 11R-HO-1 Protein in a Rat SAH Model

Microscopic examination of the BA proved efficient transduction into the arterial wall. The arterial diameter in the 11R-HO-1 injection group was significantly larger than in the control groups.

Discussion

As we mentioned above, the protein transduction method allows various proteins to be transported directly and effectively into all kinds of cells [3, 4, 6, 15, 16]. We also proved in a previous study that the marker protein enhanced green fluorescent protein (EGFP) fused to 11R has a strong transduction efficacy in rat cerebral arteries [10, 11]. Therefore, we tried to apply a real therapeutic protein to this new and apparently efficient method and could prove in the present study that 11R fused HO-1 protein has low cytotoxicity. Moreover, the protein markedly inhibited the vasoconstriction of the rat BA after SAH. Thus, the 11R-HO-1 protein transduction method can overcome the problems of gene therapy as described above and be one of the most excellent therapies in the research area of cerebral vasospasm after SAH. We will study the effects in more detail in the animal model.

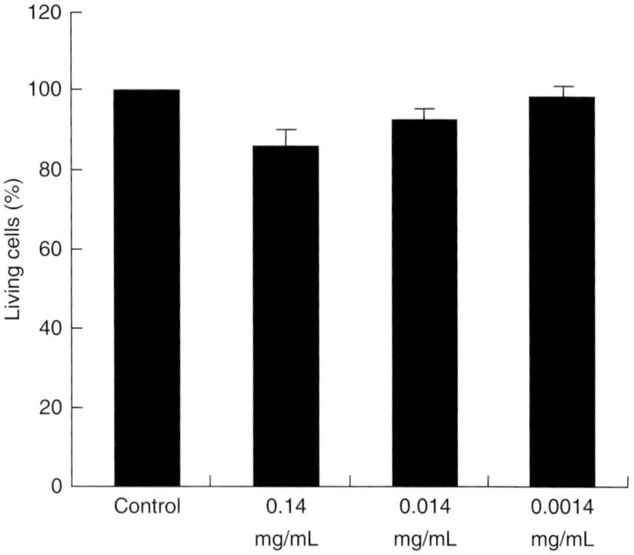

Fig. 2 Cytotoxicity of various concentrations of 11R-HO-1 protein as measured by fluorescence assay. The cells were incubated with three different concentrations of 11R-HO-1 protein (0.14 mg/mL, 1.4×10^{-2} mg/mL and 1.4×10^{-3} mg/mL) (n=7, each) at 37°C for 24 h. This graph shows that 11R-HO-1 has little toxicity at each concentration. Data are mean±SD. Concentrations of 11R-HO-1 protein and metabolic activity compared to control were 0.14 mg/mL (82.34±7.39%, n=7), 1.4×10^{-2} mg/mL (92.31±6.25%, n=7) and 1.4×10^{-3} mg/mL (98.79±2.50%, n=7). The wavelength to measure absorbance of the formazan product was 550 nm. The reference wavelength was 655 nm

Acknowledgments Dr. Ogawa is an Alexander von Humboldt fellow and the current studies were partially financed by the Alexander von Humboldt Foundation.

Conflict of interest statement We declare that we have no conflict of interest.

References

1. Chen AFY, Jiang S-W, Crotty TB, Tsutsui M, Smith LA, O'Brien T, Katusic ZS (1997) Effects of in vivo adventitial expression of recombinant endothelial nitric oxide synthase gene in cerebral arteries. Proc Natl Acad Sci USA 94:12568–12573
2. Christenson SD, Lake KD, Ooboshi H (1998) Adenovirus-mediated gene transfer in vivo to cerebral blood vessels and perivascular tissue in mice. Stroke 29:1411–1416
3. Elliott G, O'Hare P (1997) Intercellular trafficking and protein delivery by a herpes virus structural protein. Cell 88(2): 223–233
4. Frankel AD, Pabo CO (1988) Cellular uptake of the Tat protein from human immunodeficiency virus. Cell 55:1189–1193
5. Inoue M, Tomizawa K, Matsushita M, Yun-Fei Lu, Yokoyama T, Yanai H, Takashima A, Kumon H, Matsui H (2006) p53 Protein transduction therapy: successful targeting and inhibition of the growth of the bladder cancer cells. Eur Urol 49:161–168
6. Marton LS, Wang X, Kowalczuk A, Zhang ZD, Windmeyer E, Macdonald RL (2000) Effects of hemoglobin on heme oxygenase gene expression and viability of cultured smooth muscle cells. Am J Physiol Heart Circ Physiol 279(5):H2405–H2413
7. Matsui H, Tomizawa K, Lu YF, Matsushita M (2003) Protein therapy: in vivo protein transduction by polyarginine (11R) PTD and subcellular targeting delivery. Curr Protein Pept Sci 4(2):151–157
8. Matsushita M, Tomizawa K, Moriwaki A, Li ST, Terada H, Matsui H (2001) A high-efficiency protein transduction system demonstrating the role of PKA in long-lasting long-term potentiation. J Neurosci 21(16):6000–6007
9. Michiue H, Tomizawa K, Wei F-Y, Matsushita M, Yun-Fei Lu, Ichikawa T, Tamiya T, Date I, Matsui H (2005) The NH2 terminus of Influenza virus hemagglutinin-2 subunit peptides enhances the antitumor potency of polyarginine-mediated p53 protein transduction. J Biol Chem 280(9):8285–8289
10. Ogawa T, Ono S, Ichikawa T, Arimitsu S, Onoda K, Tokunaga K, Sugiu K, Tomizawa K, Matsui H, Date I (2007) Novel protein transduction method by using 11R – an effective new drug delivery system for the treatment of cerebrovascular diseases. Stroke 38(4):1354–1361
11. Ogawa T, Ono S, Ichikawa T, Arimitsu S, Onoda K, Tokunaga K, Sugiu K, Tomizawa K, Matsui H, Date I (2009) Protein transduction method for cerebrovascular disorders. Acta Med Okayama 63(1):1–7
12. Ono S, Komuro T, Macdonald RL (2002) Heme oxygenase-1 gene therapy for prevention of vasospasm in rats. J Neurosurg 96(6):1094–1102
13. Onoue H, Tsutsui M, Smith L, Stelter A, O'Brien T, Katusic ZS (1998) Expression and function of recombinant endothelial nitric oxide synthase gene in canine basilar artery after experimental subarachnoid hemorrhage. Stroke 29(9):1959–1965
14. Satoh M, Perkins E, Kimura H, Tang J, Chun Y, Heistad DD, Zhang JH (2002) Posttreatment with adenovirus-mediated gene transfer of calcitonin gene-related peptide to reverse cerebral vasospasm in dogs. J Neurosurg 97:136–142
15. Schwarze SR, Ho A, Vocero-Akbani A, Dowdy SF (1999) In vivo protein transduction: delivery of a biologically active protein into the mouse. Science 285(5433):1569–1572
16. Schwarze SR, Hruska KA, Dowdy SF (2000) Protein transduction: unrestricted delivery into all cells? Trends Cell Biol 10((7):290–295, Review
17. Verma IM, Somia N (1997) Gene therapy – promises, problems and prospects. Nature (Lond) 389:239–242

Training Models for Vascular Microneurosurgery

Uwe Spetzger, Andrej von Schilling, Till Brombach, and Gerd Winkler

Abstract *Introduction*: The number of microsurgical clippings of cerebral aneurysms is continuously decreasing. This will lead to fewer possibilities for practical training in aneurysm surgery, especially for the younger generation. Accordingly, realistic models for microsurgical training are mandatory.

Methods: We present a microsurgical setup for training on a PVC rat and on a lifelike vascular training model with specific plastic vessels (PVA), and an anatomical head as well as an experimental animal model (rabbit carotid artery bifurcation model). End-to-end and end-to-side anastomoses were performed with three different levels of difficulty and three different levels of expertise on the PVC rat model. The results of the animal bifurcation aneurysm model are also described.

Results: With increasing surgical complexity, the duration of surgery and rate of incorrect sutures of the vessel wall rise significantly. The overall patency rate of anastomosis is clearly reduced in the setup with increasing complexity grades.

Conclusion: The PVC rat model as well as the PVA vascular kit with realistic skull and craniotomy sites is a perfect tool for advanced microvascular anastomosis training. The experimental animal model represents a higher level of vascular surgery expertise and additionally is a perfect model for practicing appropriate clip application and clip occlusion of aneurysms.

Keywords Training models · Experimental aneurysms · Microsurgical training · Vascular models

U. Spetzger (✉), A. von Schilling, T. Brombach, and G. Winkler
Department of Neurosurgery, Klinikum Karlsruhe,
Moltkestrasse 90, D-76131 Karlsruhe, Germany
e-mail: uwe.spetzger@klinikum-karlsruhe.de

Introduction

Endovascular treatment of cerebral aneurysms has significantly reduced the number of microsurgical clipping procedures. This will lead to fewer possibilities for practical training in aneurysm surgery, especially for the younger generation [1, 5, 7, 10, 17, 22]. However, especially highly complex aneurysms with a wide neck will still be treated by microsurgical clip occlusion and will remain a challenge for cerebrovascular neurosurgeons in the future. Contrarily, revascularization and bypass techniques will find growing demand [21]. In view of these conditions, concepts and realistic models for microsurgical training are necessary to improve the practical skills of neurosurgeons during their training [2–4, 6, 8, 9, 12, 13, 18, 23]. We present two sophisticated plastic models that closely simulate real vascular conditions and a more complex experimental animal bifurcation aneurysm model in rabbits.

Material and Methods

We present a microsurgical setup for training on a PVC rat [14] (Microsurgical Developments Foundation, Maastricht, The Netherlands) (Figs. 1 and 2) as well as a specific vascular training model with highly elastic plastic vessels (PVA) and an anatomical head (Kezlex^{R}, Ono & Co., Ltd., Tokyo, Japan) (Fig. 3). Our highly sophisticated experimental animal model (rabbit carotid artery bifurcation model) is also described [19, 20] (Fig. 5).

In the prospective part of the study, end-to-end and end-to-side anastomoses were performed with three different difficulty levels in the PVC rat model [14]. A total of six surgeons with different expertise levels and different levels of vascular training and skills performed these surgical procedures. To reduce the surgical approach, three different types of plastic tubes were used (advanced/expert/master) to adapt the experimental setup to a scenario with different degrees of difficulty. These plastic tubes reduce the operative field and the working space consecutively and determine the trajectory and direction

T. Tsukahara et al. (eds.), *Trends in Neurovascular Surgery*, Acta Neurochirurgica Supplementum, Vol. 112,
DOI: 10.1007/978-3-7091-0661-7_21, © Springer-Verlag/Wien 2011

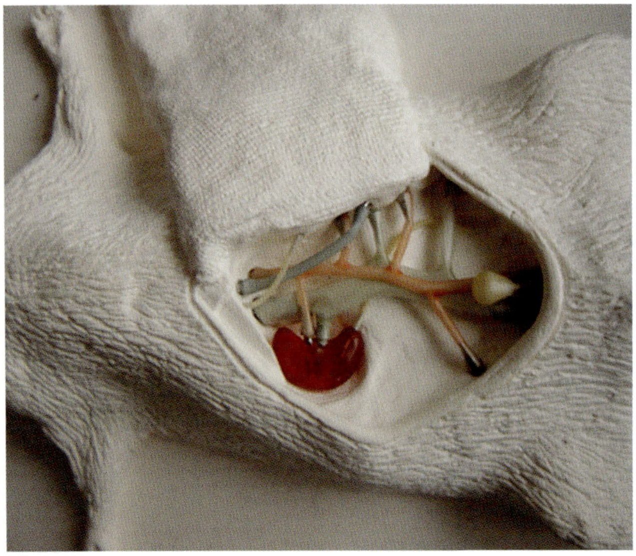

Fig. 1 Photo of the vessels of the abdominal cavity of the PVC rat (Microsurgical Developments Foundation, Maastricht, the Netherlands)

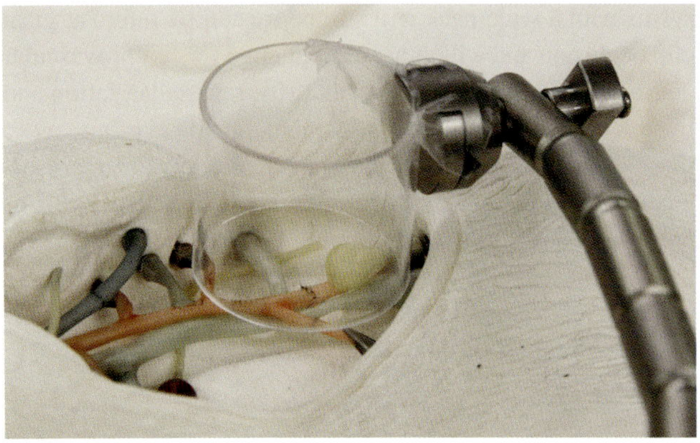

Fig. 2 The plastic tube (expert type) was fixed to a conventional flexible retractor system and reduces the working space and the operative field. In this focused working channel, the level of difficulty of performing an anastomosis increases significantly

for the instruments (Fig. 2). Because of this focused working channel, the degree of freedom to manipulate the surgical instruments is decreased, and therefore the difficulty of performing an anastomosis increases significantly. The plastic tubes were fixed to a conventional flexible retractor system (Fig. 2) and could be removed very quickly if difficulties arose intraoperatively. This is mandatory, especially if bleeding occurs in the experimental animal model. The different sized plastic tubes closely simulate intraoperative conditions in a narrow and deep surgical field. Plastic tube I (advanced) has a diameter of 4 cm and a depth of 1.5 cm. Tube II (expert) has a diameter of 3 cm and a depth of 3.5 cm (Fig. 2). Tube III (master) has a diameter of 2.5 cm and a depth of 4.5 cm. For the anastomoses we used conventional microsurgical

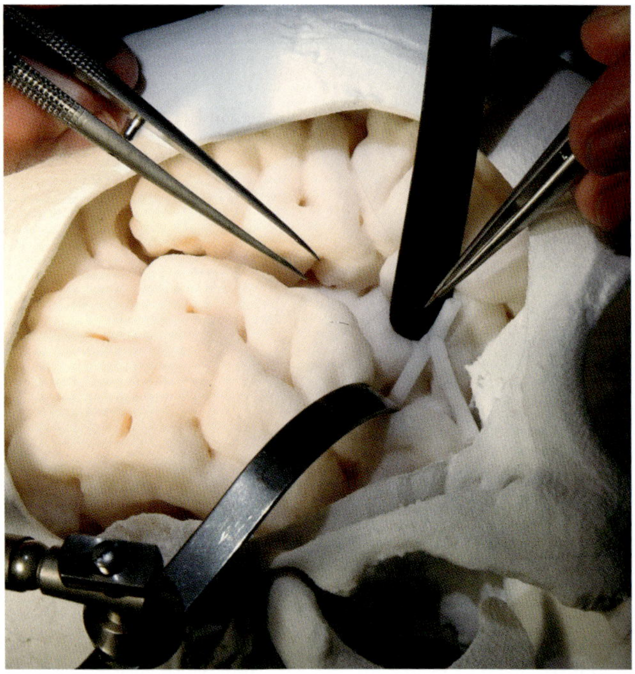

Fig. 3 The photo shows a pterional approach in the plastic skull with retraction of the soft plastic brain, opening the sylvian fissure. An end-to-side anastomosis was performed using the highly elastic plastic (PVA) vessels (Kezlex^R, Ono & Co., Ltd., Tokyo, Japan). This setup allows realistic retraction and handling of the vessels closely mimicking human conditions

instruments (S&T AG, Neuhausen, Switzerland) and monofile polyamid sutures 8/0 (BV 2) respectively 10/0 (BV 100-4) Ethilon^R (Ethicon, Johnson & Johnson Medical GmbH, Norderstedt, Germany).

Even more realistic are the plastic skull model with relatively soft and deformable plastic brain material and the vascular anastomosis practice kit with highly elastic plastic (PVA) vessels (Kezlex^R, Ono & Co., Ltd., Tokyo, Japan) (Fig. 3). The very soft and elastic plastic vessels of the vascular anastomosis practice kit are available in three different diameters: 1, 2, and 3 mm. This setup allows a realistic retraction of the sylvian fissure, and handling and preparation closely simulate human conditions (Figs. 3 and 4). The vascular kit with the humid PVA vessels gives a perfect haptic feeling during the preparation, cutting and suturing of the vessels. The whole setup with the deformable plastic brain, the realistic feeling of retraction and especially the optical impression under the microscope generate the overall characteristics of a real microsurgical human scenario. At present only few anastomoses are performed using the Kezlex^R model because of the study results based on the PVC rat model.

Material and methods of the experimental aneurysm bifurcation model in rabbits (Fig. 5) were described in detail in previous publications [15, 16, 19, 20].

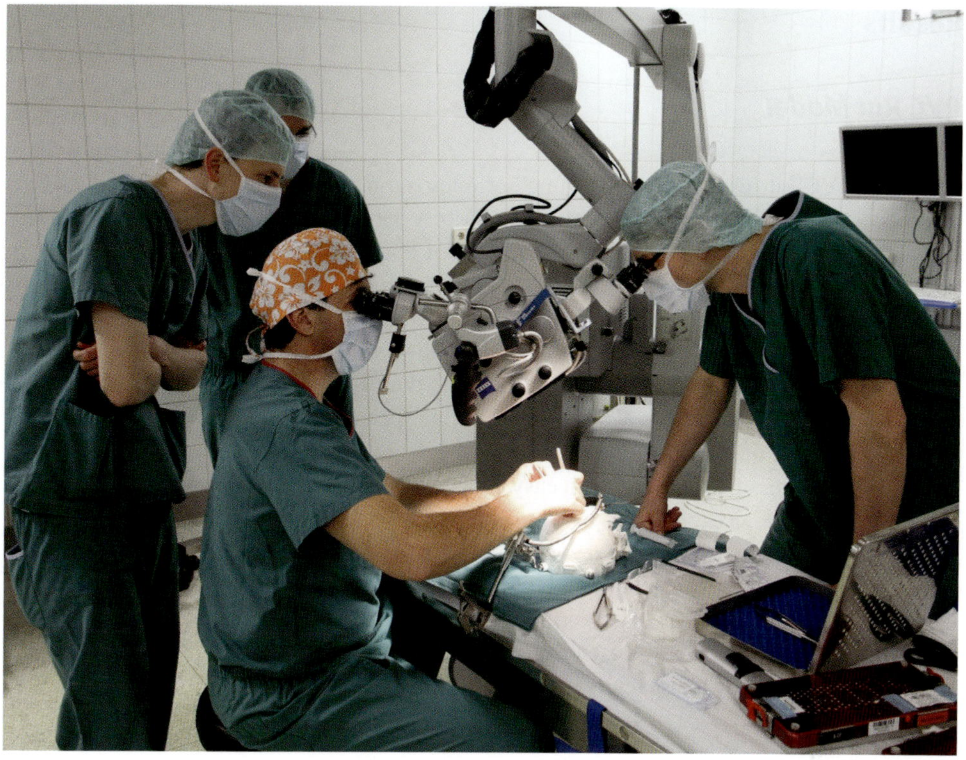

Fig. 4 Intraoperative scenario for teaching and training of microvascular surgery using different in vitro models

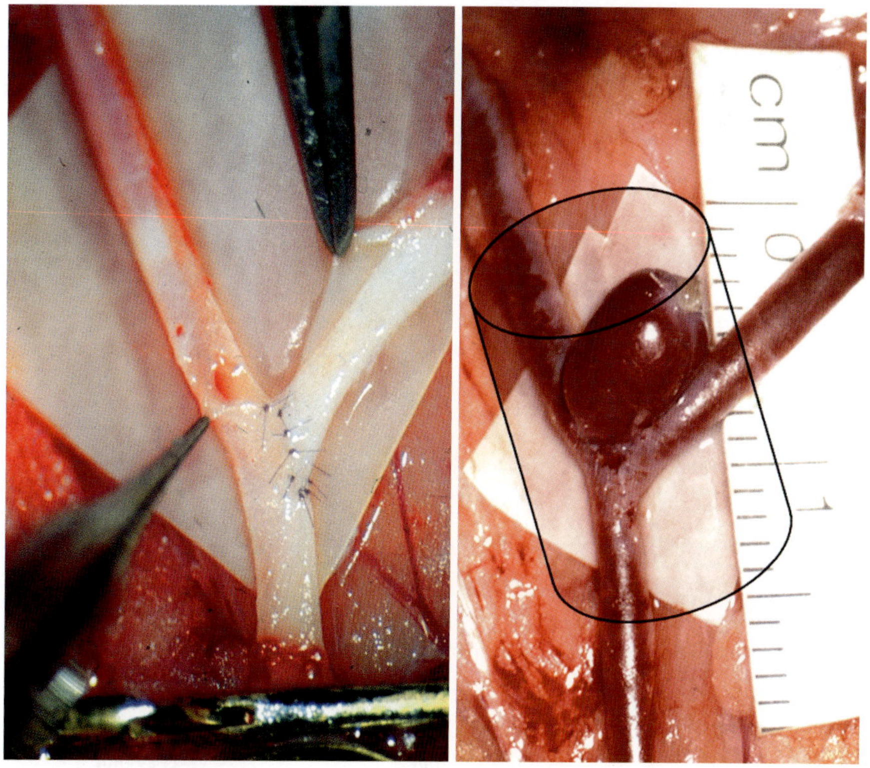

Fig. 5 The end-to-side anastomosis of both carotid arteries in the neck of a rabbit with 10/0 sutures generates an arterial bifurcation. The insertion of a venous pouch into the bifurcation then results in an experimental bifurcation aneurysm. The bifurcation aneurysm is a perfect training tool for clip application, especially if the different plastic tubes (*schematic drawing*) create a narrow and realistic working space. Because of the determined trajectory, clip occlusion of the aneurysm mimics human conditions. This setup is a sophisticated in vivo training model for active teaching and practical training of aneurysm clipping

Results

PVC Rat Model

Using the PVC rat for "unbloody training" of microsurgical techniques and improvement of practical skills is a perfect example of replacing live animals. The number of animals used in the educational training of experimental microsurgery will be reduced, and such in vitro methods facilitate the transition to in vivo models. The PVC rat model allows various microsurgical training situations, and replacing the plastic vessels is easy and relatively cheap. Using a specific nozzle at the back of the rat model, the coloured vessels can be filled with water, thus permitting an easy check of the patency and quality of anastomosis.

In Table 1 the increasing surgical complexity and reduced working space using the different sized plastic tubes clearly demonstrate that the duration of surgery and rate of incorrect suturing of the vessels rise. Consequently, the overall patency rate of anastomosis was clearly reduced with increasing grades of complexity.

PVA Vessel with Craniotomy Site

The humid PVA vessels of the vascular anastomosis practice kit are transparent, highly flexible and soft. However, they have to be kept moist and tend to dry out and lose their elasticity, especially under the high-energy xenon light of the operating microscope. At present, we use the PVA vessels of the vascular anastomosis practice kit for various experimental anastomoses. Compared to the PVC vessels in the rat model, the preparation and handling of the PVA vessels, especially grasping with forceps or insertion of the needle into the vessel wall, is more realistic and closely mimics human conditions.

The 3D model with a pterional craniotomy and the deformable frontal and temporal lobe is a perfect in vitro model to simulate an opened sylvian fissure. These realistic human skull and brain models are relatively expensive, but can be used repeatedly. However, if these models are combined and integrated, they help establish a realistic surgical scenario [11].

Animal Model

The developed and previously described animal bifurcation aneurysm model is a perfect tool for the education and practical training of microsurgical handling and preparation of cerebral vessels (Fig. 5). Additionally, it is an optimal training for bypass surgery. Additionally, this experimental aneurysm model allows optimal practical training in clip application and is a realistic teaching model for optimizing clip occlusion of cerebral aneurysms. As described in the rat model, the different sizes of plastic tubes (advanced/expert/master) were integrated into the animal model (Fig. 5). The tubes were fixed to a conventional and flexible retractor system and could be removed easily if difficulties, especially bleeding, arose intraoperatively. The plastic tubes create a narrow and deep surgical field by restricting the angle of

Table 1 Summary of the microsurgical results showing the rising surgical complexity, the duration of surgery and the overall patency rates of anastomoses

Beginner ($n=3$)	Advanced tube	Expert tube	Master tube
	Diameter 4.0 cm/depth 1.5 cm	Diameter 3.0 cm/depth 3.5 cm	Diameter 2.5 cm/depth 4.5 cm
End-to-end anastomosis ($n=6$)	Patent (75%)	Patent (42%)	Patent (8%)
	(9/12) 46 min	(5/12) 42 min	(1/12) 76 min
End-to-side anastomosis ($n=6$)	Patent (67%)	Patent (17%)	Not finished
	(8/12) 66 min	(2/12) 68 min	
Neurosurgeon ($n=2$)			
End-to-end anastomosis ($n=4$)	Patent (88%)	Patent (75%)	Patent (62%)
	(7/8) 39 min	(6/8) 31 min	(5/8) 53 min
End-to-side anastomosis ($n=4$)	Patent (75%)	Patent (100%)	Patent (37%)
	(6/8) 51 min	(8/8) 59 min	(3/8) 68 min
Expert ($n=1$)			
End-to-end anastomosis ($n=2$)	Patent (100%)	Patent (100%)	Patent (100%)
	(2/2) 15 min	(2/2) 13 min	(2/2) 19 min
End-to-side anastomosis ($n=2$)	Patent (100%)	Patent (50%)	Patent (100%)
	(2/2) 27 min	(1/2) 27 min	(2/2) 41 min

view and determine the trajectory for clip occlusion of the aneurysm just as in real aneurysm surgery. After clipping, the plastic tube is removed, and the aneurysm can be inspected easily from all sides and the clip position be checked adequately. The clip could be removed from the experimental aneurysm, and the procedure was repeated for example with a different size of tube or another angle of tube, creating a completely new situation with a different view and access to the aneurysm (Fig. 5). This is a high-end in vitro model for practical training and teaching of aneurysm clipping.

Conclusion

The PVC rat model (Microsurgical Developments Foundation, Maastricht, the Netherlands) as well as the PVA vascular model combined with the realistic brain and craniotomy site (Kezlex^{R}, Ono & Co., Ltd., Tokyo, Japan) is a perfect setup for advanced microvascular anastomosis training. The main advantages of the plastic models are the overall availability, low price and not needing a specific OR setup and instruments, as is necessary in training models with live animals. The costs and logistical considerations as well as the ethical and legal aspects involved in maintaining live animals for education and training make this relatively impractical.

The prospective part of the study with end-to-end and end-to-side anastomoses in the PVC rat model demonstrates that raising the surgical complexity significantly increases the duration of surgery and rate of incorrect suturing of the vessel wall, while the overall patency rate of anastomosis is clearly reduced consecutively.

The experimental animal model with insertion of a venous pouch within the microsurgically created arterial bifurcation is the expert training model. The resulting bifurcation aneurysm is a perfect training tool for clip application, especially if the different plastic tubes create a narrow and realistic work space for clip occlusion of the aneurysm.

Conflict of interest statement We declare that we have no conflict of interest.

References

1. Aboud E, Al-Mefty O, Yaşargil MG (2002) New laboratory model for neurosurgical training that simulates live surgery. J Neurosurg 97:1367–1372
2. Berry E, Marsden A, Dalgarno KW, Kessel D, Scott DJ (2002) Flexible tubular replicas of abdominal aortic aneurysms. Proc Inst Mech Eng H 216:211–214
3. Byrne JV, Hubbard N (2004) A novel two-stage technique for construction of experimental aneurysms. Am J Neuroradiol 25:319–321
4. Chong BW, Kerber CW, Buxton RB, Frank LR, Hesselink JR (1994) Blood flow dynamics in the vertebrobasilar system: correlation of a transparent elastic model and MR angiography. Am J Neuroradiol 15:733–745
5. Colpan ME, Slavin KV, Amin-Hanjani S, Calderon-Arnuphi M, Charbel FT (2008) Microvascular anastomosis training model based on a turkey neck with perfused arteries. Neurosurgery 62:407–410
6. Gailloud P, Pray JR, Muster M, Piotin M, Fasel JH, Ruefenacht DA (1997) An in vitro anatomic model of the human cerebral arteries with saccular arterial aneurysms. Surg Radiol Anat 19:119–121
7. Gruber A, Bavinszki G, Killer M, al Shameri A, Richling B (1997) In vitro training model for endovascular embolization of cerebral aneurysms. Minim Invasive Neurosurg 40:12–123
8. Hicdonmez T, Hamamcioglu MK, Tiryaki M, Cukur Z, Cobanoglu S (2006) Microneurosurgical training model in fresh cadaveric cow brain: a laboratory study simulating the approach to the circle of Willis. Surg Neurol 66:100–104
9. Hino A (2003) Training in microvascular surgery using a chicken wing artery. Neurosurgery 52:1495–1497
10. Kimura T, Morita A, Nishimura K, Aiyama H, Itoh H, Fukaya S, Sora S, Ochiai C (2009) Simulation of and training for cerebral aneurysm clipping with 3-dimensional models. Neurosurgery 65:719–725
11. Mori K, Yamamoto T, Nakao Y, Esaki T (2010) Development of artificial cranial base model with soft tissues for practical education: technical note. Neurosurgery 66:339–341
12. Naggara O, Darsaut TE, Salazkin I, Soulez G, Guilbert F, Roy D, Weill A, Gevry G, Raymond J (2010) A new canine carotid artery bifurcation aneurysm model for the evaluation of neurovascular devices. Am J Neuroradiol 31:967–971
13. Olabe J, Olabe J, Sancho V (2009) Human cadaver brain infusion model for neurosurgical training. Surg Neurol 72:700–702
14. Remie R (2001) The PVC-rat and other alternatives in microsurgical training. Lab Anim 30:48–52
15. Reul J, Weis J, Spetzger U, Konert T, Fricke C, Thron A (1997) Long-term angiographic and histopathologic findings in experimental aneurysms of the carotid bifurcation embolized with platinum and tungsten coils. Am J Neuroradiol 18:35–42
16. Reul J, Spetzger U, Weis J, Sure U, Gilsbach JM, Thron A (1997) Endovascular occlusion of experimental aneurysms with detachable coils: influence of packing density and perioperative anticoagulation. Neurosurgery 41:1160–1165
17. Scholz M, Mücke T, Düring M, Pechlivanis I, Schmieder K, Harders AG (2008) Microsurgically induced aneurysm models in rats, part I: techniques and histological examination. Minim Invasive Neurosurg 51:76–82
18. Senior MA, Southern SJ, Majumder S (2001) Microvascular simulator – a device for micro-anastomosis training. Ann R Coll Surg Engl 83:358–360
19. Spetzger U, Reul J, Weis J, Bertalanffy H, Thron A, Gilsbach JM (1996) Microsurgically produced bifurcation aneurysms in a rabbit model for endovascular coil embolization. J Neurosurg 85:488–495
20. Spetzger U, Reul J, Weis J, Bertalanffy H, Gilsbach JM (1998) Endovascular coil embolization of microsurgically produced experimental bifurcation aneurysms in rabbits. Surg Neurol 49:491–494
21. Streefkerk HJ, Bremmer JP, van Weelden M, van Dijk RR, de Winter E, Beck RJ, Tulleken CA (2006) The excimer laser-assisted nonocclusive anastomosis practice model: development and application of a tool for practicing microvascular anastomosis techniques. Neurosurgery 58:148–156
22. Sugiu K, Martin JB, Jean B, Gailloud P, Mandai S, Ruefenacht DA (2003) Artificial cerebral aneurysm model for medical testing, training, and research. Neurol Med Chir (Tokyo) 43:69–72
23. Tellioglu AT, Eker E, Cimen K, Comert A, Karaeminogullari G, Tekdemir I (2009) Training model for microvascular anastomosis. J Craniofac Surg 20:238–239

Surgical and Endovascular Therapy of Brain AVM

How to Deal with Incompletely Treated AVMs: Experience of 67 Cases and Review of the Literature

M. Reitz, N.O. Schmidt, Z. Vukovic, U. Grzyska, H. Zeumer, M. Westphal, and J. Regelsberger

Abstract *Introduction*: Despite the availability of multimodal treatment options, some arteriovenous malformations remain difficult to treat, either for intrinsic reasons at initial presentation or for reasons evolving during the course of treatment. Frequently, such cases can be easily resolved with further therapy, but some become a continuously growing treatment dilemma while exhausting dwindling therapeutic options.

Patients and methods: A retrospective analysis was performed to identify patients with cerebral AVM who were treated unsuccessfully. Treatment was termed "not successful" if (1) postoperative angiography showed a residual AVM or missing flow reduction after palliative embolization, (2) therapy was associated with a substantial deterioration of existing neurological deficits or death, or (3) rebleeding from residual AVM occurred after therapy. Special interest was focused on the angiographic appearance of residual AVMs, their characteristic features, and their follow-up regarding second and third therapies.

Results: According to these criteria we identified 46 internal patients from our own series of 474 patients and 21 external patients who were referred from other institutions or sought a second opinion after incomplete treatment elsewhere. Out of those 67 cases, 50 patients (74.6%) were diagnosed with a residual AVM. Eleven patients (16.4%) experienced a deterioration of their clinical condition under therapy. Six patients did not show a flow reduction after palliative embolization. Twenty-five of the 67 patients were readmitted because of an ICH, either originating from an AVM residual or under palliative embolization. Thus, an increased risk of re-hemorrhage was found for palliative embolization ($n=16$) in partially treated lesions ($n=10$) and in patients with AVM grade IV and V located in eloquent regions ($n=22$). In dealing with residual AVMs, microsurgical resection alone or in combination was found to be the most efficient therapeutic option, being successful in 58.9% of cases.

Conclusion: An estimated 10% of AVM treatments may fail because of inadequate selection of either patients or management. Besides, for thorough decision-making, angiographic follow-up in all AVM patients is mandatory to allow an early identification of patients with an incompletely treated AVM requiring a second attempt. Major attention should be focused especially on high-risk subgroups with complex AVMs, partially treated AVMs, or those treated by only a palliative regimen.

Keywords AVM · Cerebral arteriovenous malformation · Failed therapy

Abbreviations

DSA	Digital subtraction angiography
ICH	Intracerebral hemorrhage
IVH	Intraventricular hemorrhage
MRI	Magnetic resonance imaging
SM grade	Spetzler Martin grade

Introduction

Despite the availability of multimodal treatment options, some arteriovenous malformations remain difficult to treat, either for intrinsic reasons at initial presentation or for reasons evolving during the course of treatment, leading to an incomplete treatment result after the initial approach. Frequently, such cases can be easily resolved with further therapy, but some patients become a continuously growing treatment dilemma while exhausting dwindling therapeutic options. For the purpose of this study, we differentiate the term "incomplete treatment" according to the intended goal of the procedure, which will naturally vary according to the initial presentation.

M. Reitz (✉), N.O. Schmidt, Z. Vukovic, M. Westphal, and J. Regelsberger
Department of Neurosurgery, Medical Center Hamburg Eppendorf, University Hospital Hamburg Eppendorf, Martinistr. 52, 20146 Hamburg, Germany
e-mail: mareitz@uke.uni-hamburg.de

U. Grzyska and H. Zeumer
Department of Neuroradiology, Medical Center Hamburg Eppendorf, University Hospital Hamburg Eppendorf, Hamburg, Germany

T. Tsukahara et al. (eds.), *Trends in Neurovascular Surgery*, Acta Neurochirurgica Supplementum, Vol. 112,
DOI: 10.1007/978-3-7091-0661-7_22, © Springer-Verlag/Wien 2011

Decision-making for AVM treatment has to assess the natural course of untreated AVMs against the risk of treatment [15]. Currently, an international randomized controlled trial (ARUBA) is underway to clarify whether patients with an unruptured AVM really benefit from an interventional treatment or experience an inconspicuous clinical course justifying a wait-and-see strategy [26]. At present, our knowledge is still based on AVM bleeding and rebleeding rates derived from single-institution studies or statistical enquiries [1, 9, 17]. The annual risk of hemorrhage due to a cerebral AVM is estimated to range between 2% and 4% [5, 22]. In AVMs that have become clinically apparent because of hemorrhage, the annual risk of rebleeding increases up to 18% [20]. Based on hospital survival cohorts, morbidity and mortality rates range between 16%–45% and 1%–20%, respectively [2, 6, 16]. AVM therapy today is justified by the poor outcome associated with its rupture [5, 20]. Complete removal of the pathology by surgical resection alone or elimination of the arteriovenous blood flow by embolization or radiosurgery are reported to be the most effective approaches in the majority of cases. Surgical resection is associated with a mortality rate of about 3% and morbidity varying from 1% to 19% [7, 10]. Endovascular treatment is associated with mortality rates of 1–7.5% and morbidity between 0.4%–12.5% [3, 4]. Radiosurgery shows a peri-interventional morbidity of about 6–11%, with the mortality rate mainly associated with bleeding events during intervention of about 7% [13, 21]. Multimodal strategies like endovascular reduction of arteriovenous shunting followed by surgery or radiosurgery are implemented in more complex cases. All of these treatment options depend on the size, location, and architecture of the lesion, and are driven by personal and institutional experiences [25]. Clear guidelines are not available because individual aspects of the patient and the pathology can at best be fitted into rough cohorts, which for many individual cases do not allow a prediction of treatment success. Our study was focused on unsuccessful AVM treatment tracing the clinical course of these patients, identifying the reasons for failure and scrutinizing our own decision-making.

Patients and Methods

A retrospective analysis of our AVM data bank was performed to identify patients with cerebral AVM who were treated unsuccessfully at a tertiary referral center recruiting patients nationwide between 1990 and 2008. Patients were included if the primary diagnosis was confirmed by conventional cerebral angiography, and if primary treatment was performed at our department or if they were admitted for a second opinion. Treatments included (1) microsurgical resection, (2) combined treatment of embolization and surgical resection, (3) palliative embolization, (4) curative embolization, and (5) radiosurgery.

Treatment was termed "not successful" if (a) postoperative angiography showed a residual AVM, (b) therapy was associated with a substantial deterioration of existing neurological deficits or death, or (c) rebleeding due to a residual AVM occurred after therapy. Patients were not included if postinterventional angiography confirmed a complete elimination of the AVM and no signs of residual AVM were seen, or if therapeutic goals, e.g., blood flow reduction following palliative embolization seen by an increased transit time of blood flow or/and diminished size of AVM, were confirmed angiographically. Analyzing the data, the gender and age of the patients, size and location of the AVM according to the Spetzler-Martin (SM) scale, source and time of follow-up, as well as the individual courses of the patients were correlated to the treatment modality. Special interest was focused on the angiographic appearance of residual AVMs, their characteristic features, and their follow-up regarding second and third therapies.

Results

Among the 67 patients meeting the inclusion criteria, 46 (68.7%) were treated at our own clinic, and 21 (31.3%) were admitted following previous initial treatment at another institution. Patients treated at external institutions were admitted because of rebleeding ($n=5$), new neurological deficits ($n=6$), or failed initial treatment requiring a second opinion ($n=10$). Overall, 36 women (53.7%) and 31 men (46.3%) with a mean age of 32.8 years (SD 13.7, median 30) were included. Thirty-one patients (46.3%) presented before initial therapy with intracerebral hemorrhage and 12 (17.9%) with seizures. Seven patients (10.5%) showed other neurological symptoms, such as aphasia, hearing loss, and dizziness, and 17 patients (25.3%) were asymptomatic.

On initial treatment, microsurgical resection was performed in 18 patients (26.9%), and 12 patients (17.9%) were treated by a combination of embolization and surgery. In 7 patients (10.4%), curative embolization was the therapeutic goal, while in 16 patients (23.9%) palliative embolization was determined to be the intended approach. Fourteen patients (20.9%) underwent radiosurgery as the primary procedure. Only one of the patients was operated on as an emergency case after presenting with an intracerebral hemorrhage (1.5%).

SM grades of cerebral AVMs at initial presentation are shown in Table 1. Overall, residual AVM was diagnosed in 50 of 67 patients (74.6%). Eleven patients (16.4%) experienced a deterioration of their clinical condition under therapy. Six patients (10%) did not show a flow reduction after palliative embolization. Intracerebral hemorrhage was the

Table 1 SM grades of cerebral AVMs at initial treatment ($n=67$)

SM grade	Surgery ($n=18$, 26.9%)	Embo. + surgery ($n=12$, 17.9%)	Pall. embo. ($n=16$, 23.9%)	Cur. embo. ($n=7$, 11%)	Radiosurgery ($n=14$, 20.9%)	Total $n=67$
I	1 (5.5%)	–	–	3 (42.6%)	–	4 (6.0%)
II	7 (38.9%)	–	1 (6.2%)	2 (28.6%)	1 (7.1%)	11 (16.4%)
III	6 (33.3%)	8 (66.6%)	6 (37.5%)	2 (28.6%)	8 (57.1%)	30 (44.8%)
IV	3 (16.6%)	4 (33.3%)	5 (31.3%)	–	2 (14.3%)	14 (20.9%)
V	1 (5.5%)	–	4 (25%)	–	3 (21.4%)	8 (11.9%)

Subgroups "palliative embolization" and "radiosurgery" showed tendentially more high-grade AVMs (SM grade of IV or V) at initial therapy compared to other interventional techniques. Patients undergoing surgery were evenly distributed with all SM grades represented, showing the majority of lesions to be graded as SM II and III. Combined treatment of embolization and surgery was performed in SM grades III and IV only. Curative embolization was only performed in some low-grade AVMs initially (I–III)

Table 2 Localization of lesions after failed AVM therapy ($n=67$)

Localization	SM grade I ($n=4$)	SM grade II ($n=11$)	SM grade III ($n=30$)	SM grade IV ($n=14$)	SM grade V ($n=8$)
Left hemisphere ($n=25$, 37.3%)	1	6	9	5	4
Right hemisphere ($n=15$, 22.4%)	2	3	7	2	1
Corpus callosum and thalamus ($n=10$, 14.9%)	–	–	6	3	1
Cerebellum ($n=6$, 9.0%)	1	2	3	–	–
Basal ganglia ($n=11$, 16.4%)	–	–	5	4	2

Localization of AVMs after failed initial therapy. High grade AVMs at deep locations (corpus callosum, thalamus, and basal ganglia) and lower grade AVMs of the cerebellum constitute an increased risk of AVM treatment failure

reason for readmission in 25 patients (37.3%). ICH occurred within hours after palliative embolization and up 216 months following radiotherapy. An increased risk of rebleeding was found in the palliative embolization group ($n=16$), in partially treated lesions ($n=10$), and in patients with AVM grade IV and V located in eloquent regions ($n=22$). Ten patients in the subgroup being treated by palliative embolization (62.5%) suffered from intracerebral hemorrhage. Fatal outcome due to ICH was seen in two patients, both occurring within a few hours after the intervention. Lesions at risk for failed AVM therapy are predominantly situated in deep brain locations (the corpus callosum, thalamus, and basal ganglia) and are associated with a high SM grade. Nine percent ($n=6$) of the unsuccessfully treated malformations were located in the cerebellum (Table 2).

Angiographic Appearance of AVM Residuals

Follow-up angiography after initial treatment was not performed in 17 of 67 (25.4%) patients either because rebleeding occurred prior to the intended control angiography ($n=11$) or MR angiography ($n=6$) was considered to be sufficient. Five patients with residual AVMs showed spontaneous occlusion on post-interventional angiography at a 46 months (mean time) follow-up (Table 3, Fig. 1). In 11 patients, regrowth of the residual AVM was seen, exceeding its previous size (Fig. 2). Seven of these patients were treated on a second attempt. In four patients no therapy could be offered because of extensive recruitment of arterialization through white matter perforators involving eloquent brain regions. In the majority of 34 patients, the findings of an AVM residual were matching with the initial angiography. These patients were found to be good candidates for a second treatment approach. The mean time between primary treatment and diagnosis of an AVM residual was 26.3 months, with the earliest diagnosis of a residual AVM after 1 month, the latest after 96 months.

Second Therapy

Two patients were admitted with fatal rebleeding, preventing a reasonable second approach. Forty-one patients (63.1%) were treated in a second intervention. In 24 patients (36.9%) no further treatment was offered when detecting the AVM residual. In these cases, therapy was either judged to increase

Table 3 Spontaneous occlusion of residual AVM ($n=5$)

	Age (years) and sex	Localization of the AVM	SM grade	Initial therapy	ICH before therapy	ICH after therapy	Occlusion after months
Patient 1	19, F	Right frontal	III	OP	+	–	69
Patient 2	36, M	Left occipital	II	OP	+	–	17
Patient 3	15, F	Right precentral	III	Embo. + OP	–	–	54
Patient 4	8, F	Left temporal	II	OP	–	–	34
Patient 5	33, F	Left frontal	II	OP	+	–	56

In 5 of the patients (7.5%) with an incomplete treatment of a cerebral AVM after initial therapy, a spontaneous occlusion of the AVM occurred. Mean time until occlusion was 46 months. All patients were treated surgically (in one case with presurgical embolization); all of the AVMs were SM grade II or III

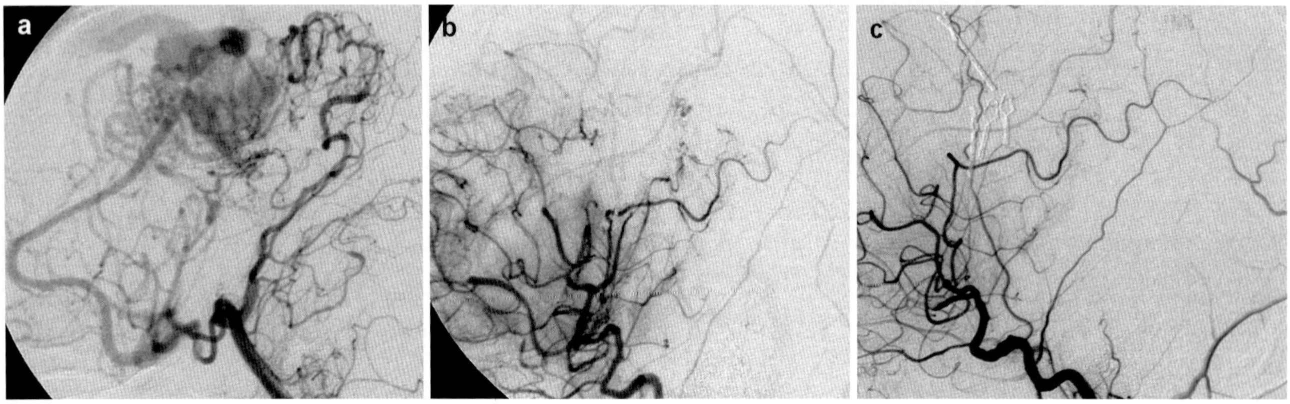

Fig. 1 Case of a residual AVM, SM grade III, in a 15-year-old female patient with spontaneous thrombosis [preoperative status shown in (**a**)]. After two-step embolization and surgical resection angiographically residual AVM (**b**). Spontaneous thrombosis was angiographically proven after 54 months (**c**)

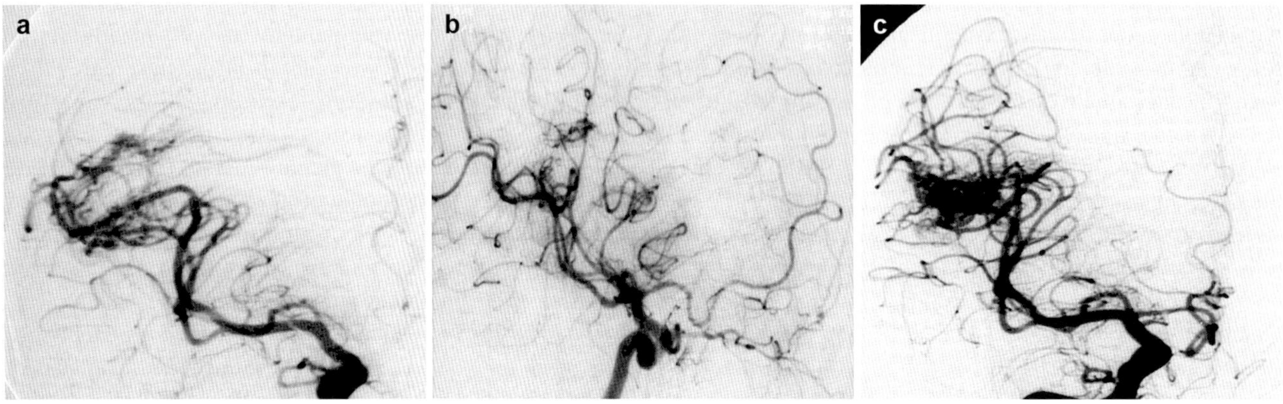

Fig. 2 Regrowth of an incompletely treated left temporal AVM, SM grade III, in a 37-year-old female. Preoperative status in (**a**), residual AVM shown 3 months postoperatively after single-step embolization and surgery in (**b**). Angiography 6 months postoperatively (**c**) reveals substantial regrowth and arterialization of the residual AVM

the risks for ICH and to be associated with a disproportional risk of neurological worsening, or control angiography showed a reduction in size of the residual AVM, warranting a wait-and-see strategy. Fourteen patients (34.1%) underwent surgery alone, and in three cases (7.3%) combined endovascular and surgical treatment was performed. Palliative ($n=6$) and curative ($n=5$) embolization as well as radiosurgery ($n=13$) was chosen for the other patients.

In eight patients (19.5%) it was possible to achieve a complete cure; all of these patients were treated by surgery ($n=7$), alone or in combination with endovascular embolization ($n=1$). In 33 patients (80.5%) secondary treatment was not successful, and treatment goals of complete elimination or flow reduction were missed. The SM grades for those AVMs being treated in a second intervention are shown in Table 4.

Table 4 SM grades of cerebral AVMs at second treatment ($n=41$)

SM grade	Surgery ($n=14$, 34.1%)	Embo. + surgery ($n=3$, 7.3%)	Pall. embo. ($n=6$, 14.6%)	Cur. embo. ($n=5$, 12.2%)	Radiosurgery ($n=13$, 31.7%)	Total ($n=41$)
I	2 (14.3%)	–	–	2 (40%)	–	4 (9.8%)
II	3 (21.4%)	–	–	1 (20%)	–	4 (9.8%)
III	7 (50%)	1 (33.3%)	3 (50%)	2 (40%)	8 (61.5%)	21 (51.2%)
IV	2 (14.3%)	2 (66.6%)	2 (33.3%)	–	2 (15.4%)	8 (19.5%)
V	–	–	1 (16.6%)	–	3 (23.1%)	4 (9.8%)

An increasing fraction of patients with high grade AVMs was treated radiosurgically after failed therapy. Eight patients (19.5%) could be treated successfully; all underwent surgical resection (in one case after endovascular embolization)

Tertiary Therapy

Ten patients were referred to a third therapy. Five patients were treated surgically, of whom three could be completely cured by total resection (Fig. 3). One patient was successfully treated by curative embolization following two surgeries. The remaining four patients are still in therapeutic planning so the final results are missing. Overall, surgery was successful on the second and third therapies in 11 patients (57.9% of surgically treated patients after initially failed therapy), thus providing the most promising therapeutic option even after repeatedly failed AVM therapy.

Discussion

To our knowledge, this is the first study in the literature focusing on failed AVM therapy, which includes the complete spectrum of therapeutic approaches. This single-center

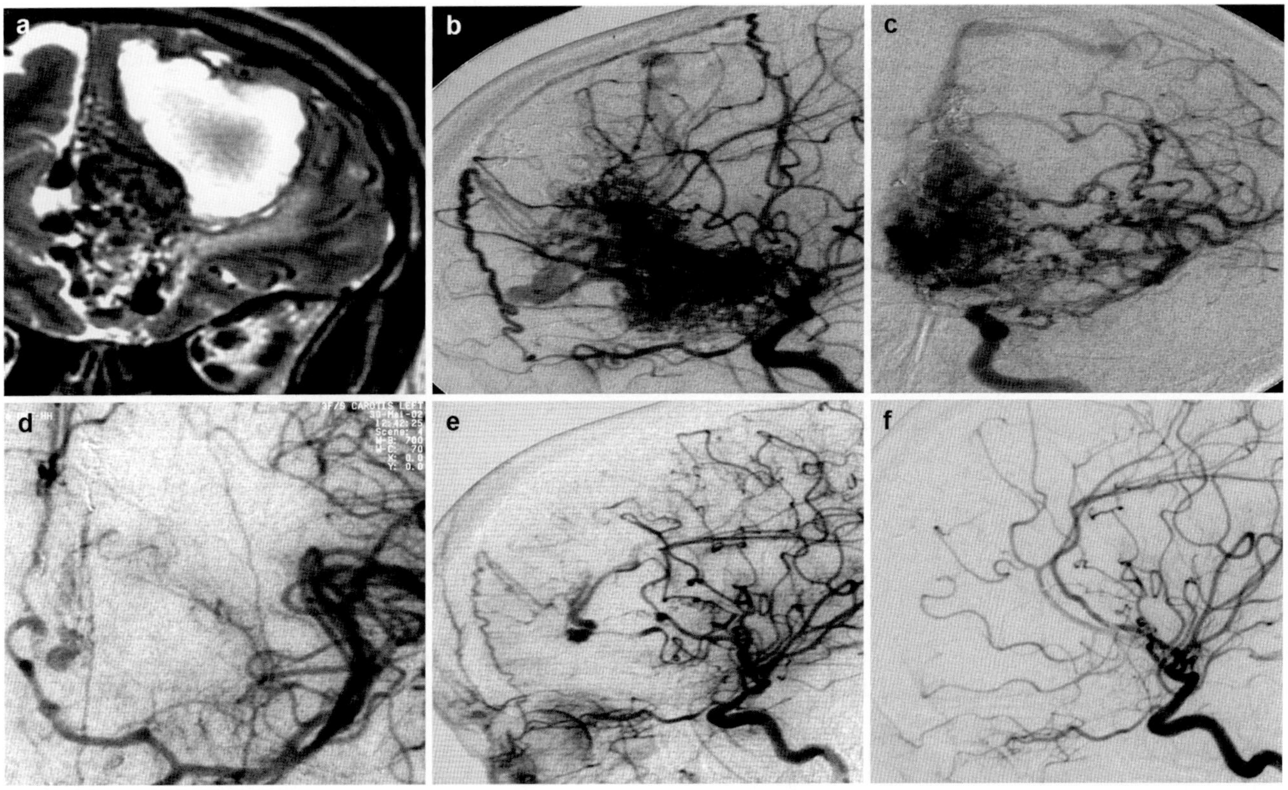

Fig. 3 Complex left frontal AVM associated with a fistulous component in a 30-year-old female. Multiple embolizations (**a–c**) were initiated to diminish arteriovenous blood flow, but the AVM was shown to recruit more arterial feeders over years. Five years after initial therapy, intracerebral hemorrhage necessitated urgent surgical evacuation of the hematoma followed by embolization and removal of the AVM (single-step) after stabilization of the patients' clinical condition. Control angiography still revealed a fistulous component of the AVM (**d**, **e**) that was surgically treated again in a successful third approach (**f**)

review, including our own patients (68.7%) as well as patients treated previously elsewhere (31.3%), was initiated to collect patients who are at risk of therapy failure and to elucidate basic principles in AVM diagnosis and treatment.

Data for incomplete microsurgical resection vary according to size, angioarchitecture and personal experience of the surgeon, but are estimated to range between 1%–18% [12, 19, 24]. However, cases of incomplete resection are the least problematic as they can be dealt with in a straightforward manner by second-look surgery. The reasons for incomplete resection are usually manifold, thus illustrating the many pitfalls associated with AVM treatment: compartmentalization (angiographically silent compartments), underestimation of the size and shape because of insufficient imaging, diffuse nidus, small AVM size, disrupted nidus after hemorrhage, and associated dural arteriovenous fistula [23].

The key point in AVM therapy lies within the therapeutic decision-making where individual aspects of the patient and lesion itself are decisive, but successful therapy is far from being predictable [28]. About 9.7% (of a total number of 474 treated AVMs) of the patients in our own AVM series were diagnosed as having an incompletely treated AVM. Our experiences have changed our treatment policy on AVM treatment, leading to a paradigm shift in the last 5 years in which SM grade IV and V patients have been treated rarely ($n=4$). Overall, surgery on the second and third therapy was successful in 11 patients (57.9%) in our series. Many of the patients initially undergoing incomplete microsurgical resection are historic and will become eliminated because of much better intraoperative imaging, such as high-resolution ultrasound and intraoperative fluorescence angiography (which is better than intraoperative DSA because of the synchronous view). Nevertheless, very small cerebellar AVMs situated in the wall of a hemorrhage, operated on in the sitting position, may remain problematic because of technical issues with ultrasound and angiography. Care has to be taken not to misinterpret early postoperative hemodynamic changes, such as reactive hyperemia due to impaired autoregulation [27]. Therefore the timing of control angiograms is worth considering on an individual basis, as is already electively planning on two postoperative angiograms to obtain two time points because an initial, early postoperative blush can either disappear or "mature" to a full AVM. In our experience, the first angiography at 3 months postoperatively will reliably confirm a residual AVM.

The majority of patients at risk of failed AVM therapy presented with high SM grades (grade III: 44.8%; grades IV and V: 32.8%), confirming the results of other series [11, 18]. We found an increased risk for postinterventional ICH following palliative embolization, which was attributed to the higher SM grades. Further risk factors for therapy failure may be deeply located lesions, partially treated AVM, and AVMs in which combined regimens are needed.

Although angiography is still accepted to be the gold standard in diagnosing an AVM, surprisingly it is not performed routinely following an AVM treatment. MR angiography is meant to be sufficient in a proportion of patients, but carries a high risk of false-negative findings [14]. Our study has shown that there are a large number of therapy failures and that an early diagnosis of a residual AVM only facilitates a targeted second therapy on time before arterialization through white matter perforators is initiated or an opening of collaterals occurs. Consequently, we strongly emphasize the necessity of a 3-month postoperative angiography in order to detect residual AVM early, thereby minimizing the risk of rebleeding by conducting a second intervention on time. A further 6- and 12-month control may be dependent on patient age, treatment modality, and preceding angiographic findings. Hyperemic, slow-flow angiomas or venous drainages suspicious of a residual AVM have to be controlled closed-meshed, because spontaneous thrombosis as well as rapid regrowth may occur. Especially patients younger than 20 years are reported to be at risk of true recurrence or early regrowth of a residual AVM. Palliative treatments are chosen to diminish the risk of bleeding, but do not eliminate the AVM completely. Radiosurgical attempts will need a 2–3-year interval before angiography can definitely exclude a residual AVM [8]. Therefore, these subgroups definitely require a thorough follow-up. While AVMs often present with a complex vascular architecture, specialized centers are required where multidisciplinary approaches are available to provide the most suitable therapy for the patient and to prevent an incomplete treatment in which secondary attempts may be even more challenging.

Conclusions

Partially treated AVMs, palliative embolization, AVM grades IV and V, and deeply located lesions that may require combined regimens constitute a high risk for AVM residuals. Spontaneous thrombosis of the residual can be observed in some cases, but the rate of regrowth and rebleeding poses potential danger to the patient. Control angiography is warranted to confirm treatment success and to initiate further therapies on time. Following initially failed therapy, microsurgical excision seems to be the most promising strategy in our experience.

Conflict of interest statement We declare that we have no conflict of interest.

References

1. Al Shahi R, Fang JS, Lewis SC, Warlow CP (2002) Prevalence of adults with brain arteriovenous malformations: a community based study in Scotland using capture-recapture analysis. J Neurol Neurosurg Psychiatry 73:547–551

2. Al Shahi R, Warlow C (2001) A systematic review of the frequency and prognosis of arteriovenous malformations of the brain in adults. Brain 124:1900–1926
3. Andreou A, Ioannidis I, Lalloo S, Nickolaos N, Byrne JV (2008) Endovascular treatment of intracranial microarteriovenous malformations. J Neurosurg 109:1091–1097
4. Biondi A, Le Jean L, Capelle L, Duffau H, Marsault C (2006) Fatal hemorrhagic complication following endovascular treatment of a cerebral arteriovenous malformation. Case report and review of the literature. J Neuroradiol 33:96–104
5. Brown RD Jr, Wiebers DO, Forbes G, O'Fallon WM, Piepgras DG, Marsh WR, Maciunas RJ (1988) The natural history of unruptured intracranial arteriovenous malformations. J Neurosurg 68:352–357
6. Brown RD Jr, Wiebers DO, Torner JC, O'Fallon WM (1996) Frequency of intracranial hemorrhage as a presenting symptom and subtype analysis: a population-based study of intracranial vascular malformations in Olmsted Country, Minnesota. J Neurosurg 85:29–32
7. Castel JP, Kantor G (2001) Postoperative morbidity and mortality after microsurgical exclusion of cerebral arteriovenous malformations. Current data and analysis of recent literature. Neurochirurgie 47:369–383
8. Chang TC, Shirato H, Aoyama H, Ushikoshi S, Kato N, Kuroda S, Ishikawa T, Houkin K, Iwasaki Y, Miyasaka K (2004) Stereotactic irradiation for intracranial arteriovenous malformation using stereotactic radiosurgery or hypofractionated stereotactic radiotherapy. Int J Radiat Oncol Biol Phys 60:861–870
9. Choi JH, Mast H, Sciacca RR, Hartmann A, Khaw AV, Mohr JP, Sacco RL, Stapf C (2006) Clinical outcome after first and recurrent hemorrhage in patients with untreated brain arteriovenous malformation. Stroke 37:1243–1247
10. Choi JH, Mohr JP (2005) Brain arteriovenous malformations in adults. Lancet Neurol 4:299–308
11. Davidson AS, Morgan MK (2010) How safe is arteriovenous malformation surgery? A prospective, observational study of surgery as first-line treatment for brain arteriovenous malformations. Neurosurgery 66:498–504
12. Deruty R, Pelissou-Guyotat I, Morel C, Bascoulergue Y, Turjman F (1998) Reflections on the management of cerebral arteriovenous malformations. Surg Neurol 50:245–255
13. Flickinger JC, Kondziolka D, Lunsford LD, Pollock BE, Yamamoto M, Gorman DA, Schomberg PJ, Sneed P, Larson D, Smith V, McDermott MW, Miyawaki L, Chilton J, Morantz RA, Young B, Jokura H, Liscak R (1999) A multi-institutional analysis of complication outcomes after arteriovenous malformation radiosurgery. Int J Radiat Oncol Biol Phys 44:67–74
14. Grzyska U, Fiehler J (2009) Pathophysiology and treatment of brain AVMs. Klin Neuroradiol 19(1):82–90
15. Hartmann A, Mast H, Choi JH, Stapf C, Mohr JP (2007) Treatment of arteriovenous malformations of the brain. Curr Neurol Neurosci Rep 7:28–34
16. Hartmann A, Mast H, Mohr JP, Koennecke HC, Osipov A, Pile-Spellman J, Duong DH, Young WL (1998) Morbidity of intracranial hemorrhage in patients with cerebral arteriovenous malformation. Stroke 29:931–934
17. Hernesniemi JA, Dashti R, Juvela S, Vaart K, Niemela M, Laakso A (2008) Natural history of brain arteriovenous malformations: a long-term follow-up study of risk of hemorrhage in 238 patients. Neurosurgery 63:823–829
18. Kwon Y, Jeon SR, Kim JH, Lee JK, Ra DS, Lee DJ, Kwun BD (2000) Analysis of the causes of treatment failure in gamma knife radiosurgery for intracranial arteriovenous malformations. J Neurosurg 93(Suppl 3):104–106
19. Majchrzak H, Kopera M, Majchrzak K, Tomalski W (2005) Treatment of deep brain arteriovenous malformations. Neurol Neurochir Pol 39:95–100
20. Mast H, Young WL, Koennecke HC, Sciacca RR, Osipov A, Pile-Spellman J, Hacein-Bey L, Duong H, Stein BM, Mohr JP (1997) Risk of spontaneous haemorrhage after diagnosis of cerebral arteriovenous malformation. Lancet 350:1065–1068
21. Nataf F, Ghossoub M, Schlienger M, Moussa R, Meder JF, Roux FX (2004) Bleeding after radiosurgery for cerebral arteriovenous malformations. Neurosurgery 55:298–305
22. Ondra SL, Troupp H, George ED, Schwab K (1990) The natural history of symptomatic arteriovenous malformations of the brain: a 24-year follow-up assessment. J Neurosurg 73:387–391
23. Pellettieri L, Svendsen P, Wikholm G, Carlsson CA (1997) Hidden compartments in AVMs – a new concept. Acta Radiol 38:2–7
24. Pikus HJ, Beach ML, Harbaugh RE (1998) Microsurgical treatment of arteriovenous malformations: analysis and comparison with stereotactic radiosurgery. J Neurosurg 88:641–646
25. Soderman M, Andersson T, Karlsson B, Wallace MC, Edner G (2003) Management of patients with brain arteriovenous malformations. Eur J Radiol 46:195–205
26. Stapf C (2010) The rationale behind "A Randomized Trial of Unruptured Brain AVMs" (ARUBA). Acta Neurochir Suppl 107:83–85
27. Stapf C, Connolly ES, Schumacher HC, Sciacca RR, Mast H, Pile-Spellman J, Mohr JP (2002) Dysplastic vessels after surgery for brain arteriovenous malformations. Stroke 33:1053–1056
28. Zipfel GJ, Bradshaw P, Bova FJ, Friedman WA (2004) Do the morphological characteristics of arteriovenous malformations affect the results of radiosurgery? J Neurosurg 101:393–401

Clinical Relevance of Associated Aneurysms with Arteriovenous Malformations of the Posterior Fossa

Nils Ole Schmidt, Matthias Reitz, Frank Raimund, Andras Treszl, Ulrich Grzyska, Manfred Westphal, and Jan Regelsberger

Abstract The aim of this study was to determine the frequency of aneurysms associated with arteriovenous malformations (AVMs) of the posterior fossa and their relation to hemorrhagic presentation in comparison to supratentorial AVMs. We performed a retrospective analysis of 474 patients with intracranial AVMs treated in our center from 1990 to 2010. Patients were analyzed for AVM size, drainage type and their clinical course with focus on vessel anomalies including AVM-associated aneurysms. Seventeen (30%) of 57 posterior fossa AVMs versus 46 (11%) of 417 supratentorial AVMs were associated with aneurysms. In six (10.5%) versus seven (1.7%) patients, respectively, flow-associated aneurysms were the source of hemorrhage. Infratentorial location of an AVM was a significant risk factor for the incidence ($p<0.001$) and rupture ($p<0.001$) of AVM-associated aneurysms. Feeding artery aneurysms in particular represented a risk factor for hemorrhage in the overall group of AVM patients, independently of the location ($p<0.001$). The majority of patients with a posterior fossa AVM were treated by combined embolization and surgical removal within one procedure ($n=33$, 58%). Feeding artery aneurysms were excluded by endovascular coiling or surgical clipping whenever feasible. Overall treatment-associated permanent morbidity in the subgroup of posterior fossa AVMs was 11% ($n=6$) and mortality 4% ($n=2$). Posterior fossa AVMs display a significantly higher frequency of associated aneurysms of the adjacent vessels that are correlated to the high bleeding rate compared to AVMs of the supratentorial compartment. We therefore recommend aggressive AVM treatment including the exclusion of associated aneurysms as a minimal therapeutic goal whenever possible.

Keywords Arteriovenous malformation · Angioma · Cerebellar hemorrhage · Cerebellar arteriovenous malformation · Cerebral aneurysm · Feeding artery aneurysm

Introduction

Arteriovenous malformations (AVMs) of the posterior fossa are rare and represent less than 15% of all cerebral AVMs [1, 2, 6]. As highly complex neurovascular lesions within a confined anatomical and eloquent compartment, the natural history and treatment of infratentorial AVMs have a higher potential for morbidity and mortality than the supratentorial counterparts [1, 5, 13]. A thorough understanding of associated risk factors in this subgroup of AVMs is therefore essential in order to develop an individualized management strategy using multimodal treatment options.

Depending on the clinical series the overall rates of AVM hemorrhage have been reported to range from 35% to 81% with an estimated annual risk of incidental hemorrhage between 2% and 4% [2]. The location of an AVM within the posterior fossa or in deep cerebral regions seems to be associated with a higher risk of hemorrhagic events [5, 16]. Besides a deep venous drainage and the presence of venous stenosis, it has been suggested that especially aneurysms on feeding arteries of AVMs may carry an increased risk of rupture [11, 17, 22]. However, results of previous studies assessing the overall relation of AVM-associated aneurysms, including intranidal and remote aneurysms with hemorrhagic events, have been conflicting [4, 6–8, 12, 18–20]. AVM-associated aneurysms appear to occur more frequently in conjunction with AVMs of the posterior

N.O. Schmidt (✉), M. Reitz, F. Raimund, M. Westphal, and J. Regelsberger
Department of Neurosurgery, University Medical Center Hamburg-Eppendorf, Martinistrasse 52, 20246 Hamburg, Germany
e-mail: nschmidt@uke.uni-hamburg.de

A. Treszl
Department of Medical Biometry and Epidemiology, University Medical Center Hamburg-Eppendorf, Hamburg, Germany

U. Grzyska
Department of Neuroradiology, University Medical Center Hamburg-Eppendorf, Hamburg, Germany

DOI: 10.1007/978-3-7091-0661-7_23, © Springer-Verlag/Wien 2011

fossa, but available data about their rupture risk are sparse [10, 22]. The higher annual hemorrhage rate of posterior fossa AVMs, which has been reported to be as high as 11.6% [1], and the still unresolved reasons for this increased predisposition to hemorrhage underscore the need for further elucidation of the associated risk factors to guide treatment decisions.

Here, we report our single-center 20-year experience in the management of posterior fossa AVMs. In particular, we compared the incidence and rupture rate of aneurysms associated with supra- and infratentorial AVMs.

Patients and Methods

Patient Population

We performed a retrospective cohort study of 474 patients with arteriovenous malformations treated at our institution from 1990 to 2010. With the exception of emergency cases, the treatment strategy was decided in a joint neurosurgical-neuroradiological conference [21]. AVM morphology and individual patient vascular architecture were evaluated by four-vessel digital subtraction angiography and standard MR imaging. Other types of vascular malformations, such as dural arteriovenous fistulas, vein of Galen malformations or cavernomas, were excluded from this study.

Clinical Presentation and Classification

Initial clinical presentation was categorized as hemorrhagic or presence of seizures or neurological deficits. Patients with unspecific symptoms resulting in the incidental finding of an AVM were grouped together with asymptomatic patients. AVM size, venous drainage pattern and eloquence of location were assessed and ranked according to the Spetzler-Martin scale as previously described [14]. Arterial aneurysms were defined as any dilatations of the lumen >2× the width of the parent arterial vessel and further classified as feeding artery or intranidal aneurysms [11, 12]. The venous angiographic phase was screened for stenotic changes during the venous outflow phase and for aneurysmal venous dilatations, which were coded as venous aneurysms.

Hemorrhagic presentation was defined as a clinically symptomatic event with signs of fresh intracranial blood on brain imaging with topographic contiguity of the hematoma with the AVM nidus or its feeding arteries. The hemorrhage was classified as related to AVM-associated aneurysms only when imaging allowed an unambiguous attribution of bleeding to an aneurysm either by brain imaging or intraoperatively. Cases with doubtful identification of an aneurysm as the primary bleeding location were not classified as hemorrhage from AVM-associated aneurysm.

Treatment and Outcome

The results of endovascular, surgical or combined treatment were assessed by routine cerebral angiography within the first 10 days after intervention and after a follow-up period of 6 months. The clinical status was evaluated at regular neurological follow-up examinations in our neurovascular outpatient clinic. Treatment-related outcome was ranked as improved, transient or permanent whenever changes of preinterventional symptoms and/or neurological deficits occurred after treatment. Morbidity was classified as permanent when not resolved after a follow-up time of 6 months.

Statistical Analyses

The incidence of AVM-associated aneurysms and risk of aneurysm-related hemorrhage was assessed by calculating odds ratios and 95% confidence intervals. Variables examined in univariate and multivariate analyses included the presence of AVM-associated aneurysms, hemorrhage related to associated aneurysms, feeding artery aneurysms, location of AVM and the presence of high-flow/fistulous component.

Results

Clinical Features

The baseline characteristics of the study cohort are summarized in Table 1. Of the 474 patients with cerebral AVMs that had been treated at our institution, 57 (12%) had an AVM localized in the posterior fossa, predominantly involving the cerebellar hemispheres. Demographic data regarding gender and age at clinical presentation were unremarkable compared to patients with supratentorial AVMs. The most common clinical presentation was due to intracranial hemorrhage. In contrast to patients with supratentorial AVMs, none of the patients with posterior fossa AVMs presented with epileptic seizures. The majority of patients had AVMs of Spetzler-Martin grades II and III.

Table 1 Baseline characteristics of 474 patients with cerebral arteriovenous malformations (AVM)

Demographics		
Male:female	265:209	56%:44%
Mean age (range)	35 (1–87) years	
Location		
Supratentorial	417 (88%)	
Lobar	361 (76%)	
Deep/midline	56 (12%)	
Infratentorial	57 (12%)	
Cerebellar	55 (11.6%)	
Brain stem	2 (0.4%)	
	Supratentorial	*Infratentorial*
Spetzler-Martin scale		
I	102 (25%)	12 (21%)
II	98 (24%)	23 (40%)
III	134 (32%)	15 (26%)
IV	50 (12%)	6 (11%)
V	29 (7%)	1 (2%)
Clinical presentation		
Hemorrhage	154 (37%)	37 (65%)
Seizure	108 (26%)	0 (0%)
Neurological deficits	18 (4%)	2 (3.5%)
Unspecific/asymptomatic	131 (31%)	18 (32%)

Table 2 Angiographic findings and analyses

	Supratentorial	*Infratentorial*
Aneurysms (total)	46 (11%)	17 (30%)
Multiple aneuryms	12 (3%)	7 (12%)
Feeding artery aneuryms	21 (5%)	14 (25%)
Intranidal aneurysms	31 (3%)	4 (7%)
Venous aneurysms	15 (4%)	2 (3%)
Hemorrhage from aneurysm	7 (1.7%)	6 (10.5%)
Venous stenosis	14 (3%)	2 (3%)
High-flow/fistulous component	46 (11%)	9 (16%)
Univariate analyses	*Odds ratio (95%-CI), p-value*	
Risk of infratentorial location for the incidence of AVM-associated aneurysms	3.39 (1.78–6.46), $p<0.001$	
Risk of infratentorial location for the incidence of hemorrhage from AVM-associated aneurysms	6.81 (2.2–21.04), $p<0.001$	
Risk of high-flow/fistulous component for the incidence of AVM-associated aneurysms	2.05 (1.01–4.14), $p=0.043$	
Multivariate analysis	*Adjusted odds ratios (95%-CI), p-value*	
Infratentorial location	1.97 (0.51–7.59), $p=0.323$	
Presence of feeding artery aneurysms	81.04 (16.18–405.86), $p<0.001$	

Angiographic Findings and Their Relation to Hemorrhage

The angiographic characteristics and their relation to the incidence of AVM-associated aneurysms and to hemorrhagic events are summarized in Table 2. Thirty percent of patients ($n=17$) with posterior fossa AVMs exhibited at least one AVM-associated aneurysm. Multiple AVM-associated aneurysms were found in seven of these patients (12%). This is in contrast to 11% of patients ($n=46$) with supratentorial AVMs exhibiting at least a single AVM-associated aneurysm. Multiple aneurysms were found in 12 of these patients (3%). The majority of associated aneurysms with posterior fossa AVMs were aneurysms of major feeding arteries (35% versus 5% with AVMs of the supratentorial compartment). No major differences were found in the numbers of intranidal aneurysms or those of the venous outflow compartment. The angiographic presence of a high-flow/fistulous AVM component represented a weak risk factor for the incidence of AVM-associated aneurysms (odds ratio 2.05, 95% confidence interval 1.01–4.14; $p<0.043$), but we found no clear predominance of a high-flow component in either of the AVM locations (Table 2). AVM-associated aneurysms were significantly more frequent in patients with an AVM in the infratentorial location (Table 2). Hemorrhage was attributed to an associated aneurysm in 10.5% of patients ($n=6$) with posterior fossa AVMs, whereas associated aneurysms in supratentorial AVMs were the source of bleeding in 1.7% of patients ($n=7$). Univariate analysis revealed an infratentorial location of AVMs as a significant risk factor for overall aneurysm-related hemorrhage (Table 2). The presence of feeding artery aneurysms in particular represented a highly significant risk factor for aneurysm rupture (odds ratio 99.0, 95% CI 20.7–471.9; $p<0.001$). This difference remained significant ($p<0.001$) in a multivariate analysis when controlling for AVM location (Table 2), indicating that feeding artery aneurysms of posterior fossa AVMs do not have a higher rupture rate than those of supratentorial AVMs.

Clinical Management of Posterior Fossa AVMs and Associated Aneurysms

Treatment of posterior fossa AVMs was performed in the majority of cases by embolization followed by immediate

Table 3 Treatment and outcome of 57 patients with infratentorial AVM

Treatment strategies	*n* = 57
Combined embolization/surgery	33 (58%)
Surgery only	19 (33%)
Embolization only/palliative	3 (5%)
No therapy	2 (4%)
Radiation therapy	1 after partial embolization
Clinical outcome	
Asymptomatic or improved	37 (67%)
Transient morbidity	12 (22%)
Permanent morbidity	6 (11%)
Mortality	2 (4%)
Lost to follow-up	9 (16%)

surgical removal within one anesthesia (33 patients, 58%) or by surgical resection only (19 patients, 33%) (Table 3). Treatment by embolization only was done in three patients (5%) followed by radiosurgery after partial embolization in one patient. Two patients with brain stem AVMs were managed conservatively. Complete resection/occlusion was confirmed by postoperative angiography in 63% (36 patients).

Feeding artery aneurysms were found in 14 patients (25%) with posterior fossa AVMs. Exclusion from the arterial blood circulation was achieved by endovascular coiling in six patients before definite treatment of the AVM or by surgical clipping during AVM surgery in four patients. Four patients had flow-related proximally located feeding artery aneurysms that were not treated directly before AVM treatment. After complete AVM resection the patients were monitored closely by follow-up angiographies, which demonstrated regression of the flow-related aneurysms within 6 months.

Follow-up information was available on 48 patients (range 3–24 months). The majority of patients with posterior fossa AVMs remained asymptomatic or displayed an improvement of the initial symptoms after treatment (37 patients, 67%) (Table 3). Twenty-two percent ($n = 12$) of the treated patients experienced a transient worsening of symptoms, which improved and finally disappeared during the first 6 months after treatment. New symptoms or neurological deficits that persisted throughout the 6-month follow-up time were classified as permanent treatment-related morbidity and occurred in six patients (11%). Two patients died as a result of the consequences of a severe hemorrhage despite the initiation of emergency surgery.

Discussion

Recent studies suggested that AVM-associated aneurysms represent a considerable risk factor for hemorrhage [5, 17, 19]. The management of posterior fossa AVMs remains a challenge despite many technological advances and is furthermore complicated by the frequent association with AVM-related aneurysms [1, 3]. Our retrospective analysis of 474 patients with cerebral AVMs confirms that infratentorial AVMs are significantly more often associated with aneurysms and especially with those located on feeding arteries. Given the tendency of infratentorial AVMs to bleed, the extent to which AVM-associated aneurysms of this subgroup contribute to hemorrhagic presentation and whether they are possibly more prone to rupture are still unresolved issues. In our study, we found a significantly higher incidence of aneurysm-related hemorrhage with AVMs of the posterior fossa than with AVMs of the supratentorial compartment. Extending our analysis, it was revealed that especially feeding artery aneurysms represented a highly significant risk factor for aneurysmal hemorrhage, which, however, was independent of the location of the AVM. Therefore, it seems reasonable to conclude that feeding artery aneurysms of posterior fossa AVMs do not have a greater tendency to rupture than their supratentorial AVM counterparts.

In terms of demographic data, distribution of AVMs at different locations and clinical presentation, our data are in good agreement with previous reports [3, 15]. However, difference exists with regard to the number of patients with AVM-associated aneurysms. In our study cohort, we identified associated aneurysms in 13% of the overall group of 474 AVM patients, whereas Stapf et al. reported 25% in a similar study group [17] and da Costa et al. 21.4% in a subgroup of posterior fossa AVMs [3]. This variance might be the result of a different selection bias. Our study has limitations since it was performed as a retrospective analysis and the study cohort consisted mainly of treated AVM patients, leaving out those who were conservatively managed. However, our data are in line with a previous single-center study that identified 7.5% of cerebral AVM patients (45 out of 600) with concurring aneurysms, in which all AVMs had a high-flow component [19]. Although we found only a weak association of a high-flow/fistulous component with the increased incidence of associated aneurysms, our data lend further support to the theory that hemodynamic stress in feeding arteries may cause aneurysm formation [9]. Our study confirms our previous report suggesting that posterior fossa AVMs are frequently associated with flow-related aneurysms, which represent a significant risk factor for hemorrhage [22]. Despite the demanding complexity of posterior fossa AVMs in our study, the treatment-related outcome was favorable with a risk of permanent morbidity of 11%, which is comparable with other well-known clinical series (reviewed in [1]).

Taken together, we recommend an aggressive multimodal therapy to treat posterior fossa AVMs. In the presence of AVM-associated aneurysms, in particular when located on feeding arteries, we advocate the exclusion of aneurysms as the minimal therapeutic goal before or during definite treatment of posterior fossa AVMs.

Conflict of interest statement We declare that we have no conflict of interest.

References

1. Arnaout OM, Gross BA, Eddleman CS, Bendok BR, Getch CC, Batjer HH (2009) Posterior fossa arteriovenous malformations. Neurosurg Focus 26:E12
2. Choi JH, Mohr JP (2005) Brain arteriovenous malformations in adults. Lancet Neurol 4:299–308
3. da Costa L, Thines L, Dehdashti AR, Wallace MC, Willinsky RA, Tymianski M, Schwartz ML, ter Brugge KG (2009) Management and clinical outcome of posterior fossa arteriovenous malformations: report on a single-center 15-year experience. J Neurol Neurosurg Psychiatry 80:376–379
4. Duong DH, Young WL, Vang MC, Sciacca RR, Mast H, Koennecke HC, Hartmann A, Joshi S, Mohr JP, Pile-Spellman J (1998) Feeding artery pressure and venous drainage pattern are primary determinants of hemorrhage from cerebral arteriovenous malformations. Stroke 29:1167–1176
5. Hernesniemi JA, Dashti R, Juvela S, Vaart K, Niemela M, Laakso A (2008) Natural history of brain arteriovenous malformations: a long-term follow-up study of risk of hemorrhage in 238 patients. Neurosurgery 63:823–829; discussion 829–831
6. Khaw AV, Mohr JP, Sciacca RR, Schumacher HC, Hartmann A, Pile-Spellman J, Mast H, Stapf C (2004) Association of infratentorial brain arteriovenous malformations with hemorrhage at initial presentation. Stroke 35:660–663
7. Lasjaunias P, Piske R, Terbrugge K, Willinsky R (1988) Cerebral arteriovenous malformations (C. AVM) and associated arterial aneurysms (AA). Analysis of 101 C. AVM cases, with 37 AA in 23 patients. Acta Neurochir (Wien) 91:29–36
8. Meisel HJ, Mansmann U, Alvarez H, Rodesch G, Brock M, Lasjaunias P (2000) Cerebral arteriovenous malformations and associated aneurysms: analysis of 305 cases from a series of 662 patients. Neurosurgery 46:793–800; discussion 800–792
9. Nornes H, Grip A, Wikeby P (1979) Intraoperative evaluation of cerebral hemodynamics using directional Doppler technique. Part 1: arteriovenous malformations. J Neurosurg 50:145–151
10. Pau A, Cossu M, Turtas S (1994) Association of aneurysm and arteriovenous malformation on the posterior inferior cerebellar artery. Report of three further cases and review of the literature. Acta Neurol (Napoli) 16:52–57
11. Perata HJ, Tomsick TA, Tew JM Jr (1994) Feeding artery pedicle aneurysms: association with parenchymal hemorrhage and arteriovenous malformation in the brain. J Neurosurg 80:631–634
12. Redekop G, TerBrugge K, Montanera W, Willinsky R (1998) Arterial aneurysms associated with cerebral arteriovenous malformations: classification, incidence, and risk of hemorrhage. J Neurosurg 89:539–546
13. Sinclair J, Kelly ME, Steinberg GK (2006) Surgical management of posterior fossa arteriovenous malformations. Neurosurgery 58:ONS-189–ONS-201; discussion ONS-201
14. Speizler RF, Martin NA (2008) A proposed grading system for arteriovenous malformations. 1986. J Neurosurg 108:186–193
15. Stapf C, Khaw AV, Sciacca RR, Hofmeister C, Schumacher HC, Pile-Spellman J, Mast H, Mohr JP, Hartmann A (2003) Effect of age on clinical and morphological characteristics in patients with brain arteriovenous malformation. Stroke 34:2664–2669
16. Stapf C, Mast H, Sciacca RR, Choi JH, Khaw AV, Connolly ES, Pile-Spellman J, Mohr JP (2006) Predictors of hemorrhage in patients with untreated brain arteriovenous malformation. Neurology 66:1350–1355
17. Stapf C, Mohr JP, Pile-Spellman J, Sciacca RR, Hartmann A, Schumacher HC, Mast H (2002) Concurrent arterial aneurysms in brain arteriovenous malformations with haemorrhagic presentation. J Neurol Neurosurg Psychiatry 73:294–298
18. Stefani MA, Porter PJ, terBrugge KG, Montanera W, Willinsky RA, Wallace MC (2002) Large and deep brain arteriovenous malformations are associated with risk of future hemorrhage. Stroke 33:1220–1224
19. Thompson RC, Steinberg GK, Levy RP, Marks MP (1998) The management of patients with arteriovenous malformations and associated intracranial aneurysms. Neurosurgery 43:202–211; discussion 211–202
20. Turjman F, Massoud TF, Vinuela F, Sayre JW, Guglielmi G, Duckwiler G (1995) Correlation of the angioarchitectural features of cerebral arteriovenous malformations with clinical presentation of hemorrhage. Neurosurgery 37:856–860; discussion 860–852
21. Westphal M, Cristante L, Grzyska U, Freckmann N, Zanella F, Zeumer H, Herrmann HD (1994) Treatment of cerebral arteriovenous malformations by neuroradiological intervention and surgical resection. Acta Neurochir (Wien) 130:20–27
22. Westphal M, Grzyska U (2000) Clinical significance of pedicle aneurysms on feeding vessels, especially those located in infratentorial arteriovenous malformations. J Neurosurg 92:995–1001

Author Index

T. Tsukahara et al. (eds.), *Trends in Neurovascular Surgery*, Acta Neurochirurgica Supplementum, Vol. 112,
DOI: 10.1007/978-3-7091-0661-7, © Springer-Verlag/Wien 2011

Subject Index

W

Printing: Ten Brink, Meppel, The Netherlands
Binding: Stürtz, Würzburg, Germany